One smoothie a day:

365 recipes for a happier, easier and balanced life

Antonietta Russo

plant based recipes and yoga asanas for the perfect lifestyle

INDEX

ONE SMOOTHIE A DAY:
introduction

Hello everyone,

and welcome to this inspirational journey. I will be with you and we will walk together through this 365 recipes for a healthier and happier life. I love smooth my meal because it is so much easier for my stomach to digest; because I feel full afterwards but yet light; because it taste great; because it push me to be more aware of what I am eating, of the way I am treating my body, my temple; because it uplift my mood with lots of different colours to play with; because I take the best that nature has to offer and I turn it into a delicious meal/snack/side/midnight crises; because it is full of the nutrient that your body needs….and kids love them!

The advantages of have a smoothies lifestyle are many. The above are just the tip of the iceberg. But now let's go back to this book. What we will find in it:

- 365 smoothies recipes from the most basic and simple to the most original and complicated
- option to modify some of the ingredients
- The W@W FACTOR in which we dig the nutrients and the benefits of some of our natural product
- TIPS on how to simplify or make more interesting our smoothie of the day
- all vegan diet based recipes
- kids friendly options
- juices friendly options
- one week smoothie/juice challenge
- yoga poses to ease the stomach and mind into the challenge
- be your own master by creating your own ideas
- ….and a little guilty pleasure with few recipes for over 21!

It is the most comprehensive book you may ever find on the market and you will have lots of fun trying it out…. and maybe develop new ideas by yourself.

All you need is a juicer and a blender!

Don't you have those? You can find very cheap on the internet, otherwise check under the recipes and you will have juicer free alternative for your ONE SMOOTHIE A DAY!

Welcome in this new healthy and happy world.

Let's start our journey

Antonietta Russo

Do you want to know more?

Do you have new ideas you like to share with me?

Do you want to know where to find some of the ingredients?

I am here for you, in and out the book!

Follow me on

Instagram: https://www.instagram.com/antoniettacreativewriter/

Facebook: https://www.facebook.com/AntoniettaCreativeWriter/

All the information include in the W@W FACTOR are a collection of extensive researched coming from different sources. They are meant to be taken has a fun fact, a point of start, a guideline to be more informed about what we eat and how the food we introduce in our body may affect us. It is not meant to be an extensive and complete encyclopaedia on the food. I am aware that a lot more has to be said on each and every fruit and vegetable listed in this book but the aim of the book is a different one and I need to be loyal to my own purpose.

One smoothie a day:
My Favourite ten

This short section aim to describe a personalised smoothie selection that contains ten of the tastier and most interesting combination of natural earthy products. All the ideas in this book are worth to be experienced at least once in the lifetime, as I did, but I know the importance to have a safe nest where to go back to when you have no time to explore the entire book and pick the right one for you.

Try all of them and cross one of the boxes on the side of each smoothie every time you find a blend that satisfy your palate in order to be able to come back to do only your favourites one.

Cross **Yes** if you like the smoothie

Cross **No** if you think is not for you

Plus, use the section ADD YOUR COMMENT to personalise your smoothie: if you like more apple or less basil, this is where you should jot down your thoughts and be the author of your life.

Here we begin…………..!!!

N.1   <u>*A colourful day*</u>   *Yes / No*

spinach	2 handful
apple	2
mix frozen berry	½ cup
mint	~ 4 leaves

HOW TO: wash the apples, spinach and mint leaves. Place the apple in the juicer (whole or cut in quarters depends on the strength of your juicer). Add all the ingredients to the blender together with the juice of the apple and press START to blend.

TIPS: if you don't have a juicer you may always buy the apple juice but be careful to the amount of sugar and additive that those long life product tend to contain. I would rather use plain water as your liquid base for the blender and use just ¼ of the apple thinly chopped to mix with the other ingredients.

ADD YOUR COMMENT: _____

_____

_____

The Earth love *Yes / No*

acai berry	(powder 1 tbsp or frozen 1 cube)
avocado	½
banana	1
spinach	1 handful
apple	3

HOW TO: wash all the ingredients. Juice only the apples. Place all the other ingredients in the blender and press START

TIPS: use only ripe avocado and banana for a less bitter taste. If you don't have a juicer cut only ¼ of your apple and add it to the blender with a ½ cup of fresh plain water.

ADD YOUR COMMENT: _____

_____

_____

THE W@W FACTOR: *Avocado*, also known as alligator pear or butter fruit, are a stone fruit with a creamy texture that grows in warm climates. *Avocados* are native to Central and South America but they are now commercially produced in the US, Caribbean, Mexico, Brazil, Israel and Australia.

They are a great source of vitamins C, E, K, and B6, as well as riboflavin, niacin, folate, pantothenic acid, magnesium, and potassium.

Avocados are full of healthy, beneficial fats that help to keep you full and satisfied. Fat is essential for every single cell in the body. In fact, eating healthy fats supports skin health, enhances the absorption of fat-soluble vitamins, minerals, and other nutrients, and may even help boost the immune system.

Benefits of the avocado includes preventing heart diseases, improve vision, limit the spread of osteoporosis, improve digestion and reduce the chance to develop cancer. Also, the folate, present in the avocado, is extremely important for a healthy pregnancy: adequate intake reduces the risk of miscarriage and neural tube defects.

It furthermore help to decrease the risk of depression thanks to the fact that folate is involved in preventing the formation of homocysteine, a substance that can impair circulation and delivery of nutrients to the brain.

N.3   *I dare you*   *Yes / No*

tomato	1 medium size
papaya	1 medium size
spinach	1 handful
mango	½
lime zest	of 1 lime
ice	½ cup

HOW TO: wash and chop all the fruit and veg and add them to the blender. Add the zest of a lime and the ice. Press START to blend.

TIPS: this smoothie is juicer free but if you like you can peel and chop the mango and add it to the juicer (1 whole mango) and add only 4 ice cubes to the mix.

ADD YOUR COMMENT: _____
_____
_____

N.4   *the fantasyland*   *Yes / No*

passion fruit	1
strawberry	4
apple	2
honey dew melon	1 slice
ice	4 cubes
agave syrup	1 tsp

HOW TO: carefully wash and chop all the ingredients. Juice the apples and then add all the ingredients to the mixer. Press START to blend.

TIPS: add only a little of agave syrup in the blender. After have mixed all the ingredients, taste it and add more syrup if necessary.
If the juicer is not available, add water instead of the apple.

ADD YOUR COMMENT: _____
_____
_____

N.5   *the posh blend*   *Yes / No*

raspberry	1 handful
banana	1
spinach	1 handful
peanut butter	1 tbsp
lemon zest	of ½ lemon
lavender tea	1 cup
hemp protein	1 tsp

HOW TO: prepare the lavender tea in advanced (keep it in the fridge for around 30 minutes). Place all the ingredients in the blender together with the tea and press START.

TIPS: if the lavender tea is not your favourite, opt for a green tea or mix apple and carrot for a more earthy taste.

ADD YOUR COMMENT: _____

_____

_____

N.6   *sleeping beauty*   *Yes / No*

coffee powder	1 tsp
coconut yoghurt	2 tbsp
ice	½ cup
banana	½
avocado	½
ground almond	1 tbsp
ground coconut	1 tbsp

HOW TO: you only need the blender. Place all the ingredients together and press START

TIPS: add a tsp of cocoa for a sweet twist

ADD YOUR COMMENT: _____

_____

_____

N.7 <u>when the sun goes down</u>   Yes / No

fig	2
apple	2
strawberries	4
kiwi	1
lime	½
papaya	1 small

HOW TO: wash all the fruits properly, peel the figs, kiwi and papaya. Add them into the blender. Cut 1 lime in half and squeeze the juice inside the blender. Use the juicer for the 2 apples and pour the juice in the blender. Press START.

TIPS: I like to leave the leaves of the strawberries in the blender but, up to you! If you don't have a juicer simply take out the apples from the shopping list and use instead fresh plain water.

ADD YOUR COMMENT: _____
_____
_____

N.8   <u>the doctor said...</u>   Yes / No

fennel	1
cucumber	½
avocado	1
ginger	1 tsp
lemon	½
salt	a pinch

HOW TO: place in the juicer the fennel, cucumber, ginger and the ½ lemon. Pour the juice in the blender and add the remaining ingredients. Press START.

TIPS: keep your smoothie in the fridge for 30 minutes before to savour it. If you don't have a juicer squeeze the ½ lemon straight into the blender, grate the ginger, chop ½ fennel only and the ½ cucumber. Add little water.

ADD YOUR COMMENT: _____
_____
_____

N.9   _refresh me now_   Yes / No

kale	1 handful
blueberries	1 handful
dairy free vanilla ice cream	2 tbsp
ice	½ cup
banana	1
mint	3 leaves

HOW TO: wash properly the fruit and vegetables. Place all the ingredients in the mixer and blend.

TIPS: avoid the ice by adding 1 cup of soy milk and keep in the fridge for 10 to 15 minutes

ADD YOUR COMMENT: _____

_____

_____

N.10   _wonderland_   Yes / No

coconut water	1 cup
frozen berries	½ cup
pumpkin seeds	1 tsp
chia seeds	1 tsp
cashew nuts (soaked)	⅓ of a cup
kale	1 handful
banana	½

HOW TO : soaked the cashew nuts in water overnight. Add all the ingredients in the blender and press START.

TIPS: if you don't have time to keep the nuts overnight in the water, bring the water to boil and keep the cashews in it for 15 minutes.

ADD YOUR COMMENT: _____

_____

_____

One smoothie a day:
Let's Start with the Fun

This chapter it offers you 50 different smoothies idea that you can pick from every time you need inspiration. It's a mix of breakfast or lunch smoothies, sweet or spicy, fruity or veggie, easy to make or requiring an extra bit of attention.

Try all of them and cross one of the boxes on the side of each smoothie every time you find a blend that satisfy your palate in order to be able to come back to do only your favourites one.

Cross **Yes** if you like the smoothie

Cross **No** if you think is not for you

Plus, use the section ADD YOUR COMMENT to personalise your smoothie: if you like more apple or less basil, this is where you should jot down your thoughts and be the author of your life.

N.11   _fast fun_   Yes / No

green tea	¾ cup
blueberry	½ cup
banana	1
ice	4 cubes

HOW TO: prepare the green tea in advance by placing the tea bag in a cup with a tiny bit of hot water. Let it brew and add cold water until the cup is filled. Add all the ingredients in the blender and press START to mix.

TIPS: choose ripe banana for your smoothies, it gives a less bitter taste.
This smoothie is juicer free!
Remember, you are the artist, if you enjoy more a different kind of tea give it a try and discover new flavours.

ADD YOUR COMMENT: _____

_____

_____

<u>The Rich Ball</u>   Yes / No

apple	2
celery	3 stalk
banana	1
avocado	1
mint	5 leaves
spinach	1 handful
ginger	1 tsp

HOW TO: place in the juicer only celery, apple and ginger. Pour the juice into the blender together with all the other ingredients and press START.

TIPS: opt for ripe avocado and banana for a smoother and less bitter taste. Go juicer free by grating the ginger, chop only 1 celery stalk straight into the blender and use only ¼ of the apple. Add ½ cup of water.

ADD YOUR COMMENT: _____

_____

_____

The W@W factor: *Celery* is a marshland plant cultivated as a vegetable since antiquity. Its seeds are use either as a spice that in herbal medicine. The first cultivation is thought to have happened in the Mediterranean region where the salty and wet soils promote the celery growth.

Celery contains minerals such as calcium, sodium, copper, magnesium, iron, zinc, and potassium. It contains fatty acids and vitamins including vitamin A, K, C, E, D, and the B vitamins (thiamin, riboflavin, folic acid, vitamin B6, and vitamin B12). It also contains fiber. It has both antioxidant and anti-inflammatory property that help improve blood pressure and cholesterol level, prevent heart disease and protect the liver health, it boost digestion and weight loss.

Plus, contains high percentage of water and electrolytes which prevent dehydration, act as a diuretic and reduce bloating.

N.13　　　　　*red of love*　　　　*Yes / No*

beetroot	2
tomato	1
pear	2
spinach	1 handful
kale	1 handful
parsley	4 leaves
still water	⅓ cup

HOW TO: place in the juicer the beetroot and the pears. Place all the ingredients in the blender and press START to blend.

TIPS: keep adding plain still water until you reach the quantity wished for your smoothie. If you don't have a juicer, chop and place one pear and one beetroot into the blender and use a ½ cup of water.

ADD YOUR COMMENT: _____

_____

_____

N.14　　*a tale of love and war*　　*Yes / No*

romaine lettuce	1 handful
watermelon	2 slices
parsley	5 leaves
mango	1
kale	1 handful
maca powder	1 tsp

HOW TO: juice only the watermelon. Wash properly all your vegetables. Peel and chop the mango and remove the stone. Add all the ingredients in the blender and press START.

TIPS: you can make your life easier by simply buying the watermelon juice but honestly I'm against the juices pre-made because they always have some kind of additive and sugar content that are not the healthier option for your body.

ADD YOUR COMMENT: _____

_____

_____

N.15   *Surya Namaskara*   Yes / No

cold coffee	½ cup
spinach	1 handful
soy yoghurt	2 tbsp
banana	1
cocoa	1 flat tbsp
cinnamon	1 tsp
water	½ cup

HOW TO: make a long coffee with your coffee maker then mix all the ingredients in the blender and top with plain spring water.

TIPS: adjust the quantity of water and coffee following your own needs. If you are a coffee addicted add more coffee and less water. If one sip of coffee is enough to keep you awake for a week reduce the amount of coffee and increase the amount of water.

ADD YOUR COMMENT: _____

_____

_____

N.16   *anytime good*   Yes / No

swiss chard	1 handful
pecans	1 handful
almond milk	1 cup
pear	1
chia seeds	1 tsp

HOW TO: wash and chop the pear and the Swiss chard. Place all the ingredients in the blender and press START.

TIPS: add a drop of maple syrup for extra sweetness

ADD YOUR COMMENT: _____

_____

_____

<u>The awakening</u> *Yes / No*

vanilla extract	~6 drops
frozen berries	3 tbsp
coconut milk	¾ full cup

HOW TO: place all the ingredient in a blender and press START

TIPS: if you have vanilla stick use those instead by breaking a ~2 cm of stick and blend it together with the other ingredients

ADD YOUR COMMENT: _____
_____
_____

THE W@W FACTOR: *Vanilla* is a flavouring derived from orchids of the genus *Vanilla*, primarily from the Mexican, flat-leaved, species. It contains magnesium, iron, sugar, potassium, vitamin B6 and more…
It has a number of important benefits, including its ability to treat acne, improve hair growth, speed healing, reduce inflammation, prevent chronic diseases and protect the heart.

Research on the cardiovascular impact of *vanilla*, particularly its active ingredient, vanillin, has shown that it can measurably reduce cholesterol levels in the body: this is very important for people at high risk of heart attacks and strokes, as lower cholesterol can prevent atherosclerosis, inflammation in the arteries, and blood clots.

Furthermore, the smell of *vanilla* is known to directly impact the brain and induce calmness. Therefore, the extract can be one of the best and most accessible remedies for anxiety and chronic stress.

N.18   *The Breath Taken*   *Yes / No*

mint		~30 leaves
cucumber chunk	½	
strawberries	10	
ice	½ cup	

HOW TO: wash thoroughly all the ingredients. Chop the cucumber in chunks and add everything in the blender.

TIPS: make sure you have someone to kiss after drinking this smoothie because your breath will just be like heaven.

ADD YOUR COMMENT: _____

_____

_____

N.19   *a new addiction*   *Yes / No*

cherries	10
green tea	½ cup
banana	½
carrot	2

HOW TO: prepare the green tea by adding the tea bag in few drops of hot water for 3 minutes. Add then cold water. Juice the carrots and pit the cherries. Place all the ingredients in the blender and press START.

TIPS: add a tsp of spirulina to boost your energy. If a juicer is not available, proceed as before. Cut one carrot in small pieces and add it to the mix.

ADD YOUR COMMENT: _____

_____

_____

Freeze the Night   Yes / No

blueberries	½ cup
dairy free coconut ice cream	2 tbsp
lemon	½
ice	½ cup
kiwi	2

HOW TO: squeeze half lemon in the blender. Peel and chop the kiwis, wash the blueberries and add all the ingredients in the blender. Press START.

TIPS: why instead of drink it, don't you place the blend in a bowl, top with some coconut shaving and few blueberries and scoop it right in.

ADD YOUR COMMENT: _____

_____

_____

N.21   *no date no gain*   Yes / No

dates	4 pitted
spirulina mix with ⅓ cup of water	1 tsp
ice	½ cup
dairy free almond ice cream	2 tbsp

HOW TO: mix the spirulina powder with ⅓ cup of water. Place all the other ingredients in the blender and mix.

TIPS: add 1 tsp of cinnamon powder for extra flavour

ADD YOUR COMMENT: _____

_____

_____

It's a Fabulous day   *Yes / No*

carrot	5
spinach	1 handful
parsley	5 leaves
mint	5 leaves
mango	1
wheatgrass	1 tsp
ginger	2 tsp
avocado	1

HOW TO: juice the carrots and the ginger. Peel and chop the mango. Peel and scoop the avocado. Blend all the ingredients together.

TIPS: choose ripe ingredients so that the flavour is less bitter. If the juicer is not available add either plain water instead of the carrot juice or maybe try coconut water….it tastes great!

ADD YOUR COMMENT: _____

_____

_____

N.23   *I Like it Strong*   *Yes / No*

coconut fresh	2 tbsp
passion fruit	1
carrot juice	4
wasabi powder	1 tsp
pak choi leaves	3
fennel juice/chunk	1

HOW TO: juice the carrots and place the juice in the blender. Cut the fennel in half: half to be juiced, half to be diced and place both in the blender. Chop the passion fruit and place it with the rest of the ingredients.

TIPS: if a fresh coconut is not available, use instead the creamy part of the coconut milk usually sold in can. Before to open the can, let it rest in the fridge overnight.

ADD YOUR COMMENT: _____

_____

_____

The Sweet and the Spicy *Yes / No*

kiwi	2
apple	2
celery	1 stalk
pear	1
peach	1
ginger	25 ml
turmeric powder	1 tsp
red chilli (powder)	½ tsp

HOW TO: juice the kiwi, apple, celery and ginger. Add the juice to the blender together with the other ingredients and press START.

TIPS: either use turmeric powder or juice a 3-4 cm of fresh turmeric. If a juicer is not available, simply chop the kiwi and the celery and add it to the blender. Grate the ginger and add only ¼ of an apple. Top with water.

ADD YOUR COMMENT: _____

_____

_____

THE W@W FACTOR: *Turmeric* is a rhizomatous herbaceous perennial flowering plant of the ginger family. It is native to the Indian subcontinent and Southeast Asia, and requires temperatures between 20 and 30 °C (68 and 86 °F) and a considerable amount of annual rainfall to thrive. Plants are gathered annually for their rhizomes and propagated from some of those rhizomes in the following season.

When not used fresh, the rhizomes are boiled in water for about 30–45 minutes and then dried in hot ovens, after which they are ground into a deep-orange-yellow powder commonly used as a coloring and flavoring agent in many Asian cuisines, especially for curries, as well as for dyeing. *Turmeric* powder has a warm, bitter, pepper-like flavor and earthy, mustard-like aroma.

Turmeric is one of the most nutritionally rich herbs. It contains good amounts of protein, vitamin C, calcium, iron, dietary fiber, sodium, and about 24 calories in a 1 tablespoon serving of turmeric powder. It also provides a rich supply of vitamin B6, potassium, magnesium, and manganese. Curcumin is the most important active ingredient of this "super herb".

The amazing health benefits of *turmeric* and curcumin include the ability to reduce inflammation, heal wounds, improve skin health, protect cognitive abilities, and ease menstrual difficulties. *Turmeric* also helps eliminate depression, alleviate pain, slow down aging, protect the digestive tract, and prevent cancer.

N.25   A Fresh Sensation   *Yes / No*

aloe vera	½ cup
kale	1 handful
cantaloup melon	1 slice
avocado	½
dried coconut	1 tbsp

HOW TO: chop the melon and place it in the blender with all the other ingredients. Top with the aloe vera juice. Blend!

TIPS: keep the blend in the fridge for half an hour, shake it and drink it. P.S. you can also juice the melon if you like a more juicy consistency.

ADD YOUR COMMENT: _____

_____

_____

N.26   Wild Thing   *Yes / No*

green tea	½ cup
banana	1
kale	1 handful
spinach	1 handful
cucumber	½

HOW TO: prepare the ½ cup of green tea in advance. Juice the cucumber and add all the ingredients to the blender. Press START.

TIPS: the easier way to prepare a quick cold green tea is to place a tiny bit of hot water in a cup and let the tea bag sink in it. Once the flavour is strong enough for you, take the tea bag out and add more cold water until desired.
P.S. if the juicer is not available, simply chop your cucumber straight into the blender

ADD YOUR COMMENT: _____

_____

_____

Brrrrrrr......the freeze!   Yes / No

dairy free vanilla ice cream	2 tbsp
spinach	1 handful
mango	1
mint	3 leaves
ice	3 cubes
oat milk	¾ cup

HOW TO: wash properly all the veggie. Peel and chop the mango. Place all the ingredients in the blender and press START

TIPS: use any dairy free milk alternative of your choice.

ADD YOUR COMMENT: _____

_____
_____

N.28   _Beach Time, babe!_   Yes / No

coconut water	1 cup
pineapple	1 slice
kale	1 handful
fennel	3 wedges
blueberries	1 handful
agave syrup	a pinch
maca powder	1 tsp

HOW TO: wash all the fruits and the veggie. Chop the pineapple and the fennel and place it in the blender with the rest of the ingredients.

TIPS: when preparing the slice of pineapple, cut the central part out because it tends to be hard and bitter.

ADD YOUR COMMENT: _____

_____
_____

N.29   *The Choice!*   Yes / No

orange	3
passion fruit	1
pac choi	1
mint	4
ginger	a pinch
lime	½
avocado	½

HOW TO: peel and juice the oranges. Juice the ginger. Squeeze the lime juice in the blender. Wash and chop all the other ingredients and place it in the blender too.

TIPS: for this one use only the heart of the pac choi leaving the leaves out for another smoothie. If the juicer is not available, simply grate the ginger straight into the blender, add one peeled orange to the mix and add water if needed.

ADD YOUR COMMENT: _____

_____

_____

N.30   *The Rabbit Hole*   Yes / No

coriander	7 leaves
orange	3
mango	1
banana	½
raspberries	1 handful

HOW TO: peel and juice the oranges. wash and chop all the veg and fruits and place it in the blender. Press START

TIPS: add more coriander if you like a stronger taste. If the juicer is not available, simply place one peeled orange in the blender and top up with water.

ADD YOUR COMMENT: _____

_____

_____

N.31   *The Herby*   *Yes / No*

coriander	7 leaves
parsley	7 leaves
mint	7 leaves
fennel	1
apple	2
raspberries	1 handful

HOW TO: juice the apple and the fennel and then add all the ingredients in the blender and press START

TIPS: add some agave syrup to make it sweeter. If you don't have a juicer, add ½ of the fennel straight into the blender with ¼ of the apple. Top it up with water

ADD YOUR COMMENT: _____
_____
_____

N.32   *Spirulalert*   *Yes / No*

spirulina	1 tsp
coconut yoghurt	2 tbsp
ice	½ cup
mix berry	¾ cup (frozen/fresh)
acai berry	1 frozen cube

HOW TO: place all the ingredients in the blender and press START

TIPS: if you like avoid so much ice, mix the tsp of spirulina powder with a cup of spring water and use it instead of the ice as a base for your blend

ADD YOUR COMMENT: _____
_____
_____

N.33   _A Special Time_   Yes / No

mango	½
green tea	¾ cup
soy yoghurt	2 tbsp
raspberry	1 handful
lemon zest	of 1 lemon
ice	4 cubes
banana	½

HOW TO: Prepare the green tea in advance. Grate the zest out of a lemon and place it in the blender together with all the other ingredients and press START

TIPS: use either frozen or fresh raspberries, up to you!

ADD YOUR COMMENT: _____

_____

_____

N.34   _The Oasis in the Desert_   Yes / No

dates	3 pitted
apple	3
kale	1 handful
banana	1
cocoa	1 tbsp
coconut shavings	1 tbsp

HOW TO: juice the apples and place all the ingredients in the blender and press START

TIPS: a tasty option for the cocoa powder is a tbsp of chocolate shaving. If you have a chocolate bar at home don't waste it but instead shave a full spoon out of it and mix it with your blend.

ADD YOUR COMMENT: _____

_____

_____

A Balanced Life   *Yes / No*

chia seeds	1 tsp
dairy free plain ice cream	2 tbsp
spirulina	1 tsp
spinach	1 handful
turmeric powder	1 tsp
banana	1

HOW TO: mix spirulina and turmeric with a cup of cold plain spring water. Add all the other ingredients in the blender and press START

TIPS: leave the chia seed soaking in a cup with little water for 10-15 minutes before to blend to promote their natural grow.

ADD YOUR COMMENT: _____

_____

_____

N.36   _Juicer Free_   *Yes / No*

water	1 cup
banana	1 ½
kiwi	3
ice	3 cubes

HOW TO: peel and chop kiwis and bananas and place it in the blender. Add the plain still water and the ice cubes and press START

TIPS: would you like to explore a more interesting flavour? Use sparkling water instead of the still and notice the difference.

ADD YOUR COMMENT: _____

_____

_____

The power of the elements   Yes / No

flax seeds	1 tsp
chia seeds	1 tsp
avocado	1
kiwi	2
spinach	1 handful
spirulina	1 tsp
ice	5
cucumber	1

HOW TO: let the chia seeds soak in a little water for 10 minutes. Juice the cucumber. Peel and chop the kiwis and avocado. Wash carefully the spinach. Place all the ingredients in the blender and press START

TIPS: if a juicer is not available, add only ⅓ of the cucumber in the blender and top it up with either water or green tea.

ADD YOUR COMMENT: _____

_____

_____

N.38   *The Bitter Green*   Yes / No

broccoli	1 handful
kale	1 handful
apple	2
lime	½
lemon	½

HOW TO: juice apple, lemon and lime and blend with the other ingredients listed above.

TIPS: add wheatgrass powder for extra energy boost. If a juicer is not available, simply squeeze the ½ lime and lemon straight in the blender. Add only ¼ of the apple and top it up with plain water.

ADD YOUR COMMENT: _____

_____

_____

N.39   _The Plug me in_   Yes / No

orange	2
avocado	1 ½
mint	5 leaves
celery	3 stalks

HOW TO: juice the celery stalks and the oranges. Add the rest of the ingredients in the blender and press START

TIPS: play with the amount of celery to find the best balance between sweetness and bitterness in your smoothie

ADD YOUR COMMENT: _____
_____
_____

N.40   _Spring of Sin_   Yes / No

lavender tea	1 cup
mint	6
lemon	1
liquorice	1 stick (~5cm long)
banana	1 ½
ice	2 cubes

HOW TO: prepare the lavender tea in advance. Squeeze the juice of one lemon in the blender. Chop the liquorice stick in tiny pieces and add it to the mix together with the other ingredients. Press START

TIPS: you can either use the liquorice stick or 1 tbsp of liquorice powder.

ADD YOUR COMMENT: _____
_____
_____

N.41   *The Dragon age*   *Yes / No*

mint	5 leaves
watermelon	½ cup
sparkling water	¾ cup
dragon fruit	½
papaya	1

HOW TO: wash, peel and chop all of the ingredients in the blender, add the water and press START

TIPS: add a tsp of wheatgrass powder to boost your energy level

ADD YOUR COMMENT: _____

_____

_____

N.42   *The UnderGround*   *Yes / No*

potato boiled	1 medium size
broccoli	½
salt	a pinch
avocado	½
carrot	4 large
cumin seeds	1 tsp

HOW TO: boiled the potato and the broccoli in advance together with the salt and the cumin seeds. Once soft, let it cool down or run it under cold water. Juice the carrots. Place all of the ingredients in the blender.

TIPS: you may wish to add a tsp of maple syrup to the mix.

ADD YOUR COMMENT: _____

_____

_____

N.43 _The Magic Night_ Yes / No

liquorice	1 stick
papaya	1
mint	6
spinach	1 handful
green tea	1 cup

HOW TO: prepare the green tea in advance. Wash and chop all the other ingredients and place it in the mixer. Press START.

TIPS: make sure the liquorice is chopped in tiny pieces or is in the powder form (1 tbsp), unless you have a high speed blender.

ADD YOUR COMMENT: _____

_____

_____

N.44 _The Invincible_ Yes / No

potato	1 medium size
kale	1 handful
avocado	½
beetroot	3
fig	2
ice	4 cubes

HOW TO: boil the potato in advance with a tiny bit of salt. Juice the beetroot. Place all the ingredients in the blender and press START

TIPS: if a Juicer is not available, place only one diced beetroot in the blender and top it up with water.

ADD YOUR COMMENT: _____

_____

_____

**The Super weird!**   Yes / No

cucumber	1
pear	1
banana	1
kale	1 handful
ginger	20 ml
walnut	1 handful

HOW TO: juice the cucumber and the ginger. Add the juice to the blend together with the rest of the ingredients and press START.

TIPS: remember to wash your fruit and vegetable properly before to place them into the blender. And why don't you add a half spoon of protein powder to your mix to enhance the energy level?
P.S. If a juicer is not available, grate the ginger and place ½ of the cucumber in the blender. Top it up with water.

ADD YOUR COMMENT: _____

_____

_____

THE W@W FACTOR: the _pear_ tree it seems to have its origins in the Caucasus from where it spread to Europe and Asia where it was first cultivated over 4.000 years ago. Both the ancient Greeks and Romans valued the fruit for its flavour and medicinal properties.
One fresh, medium-sized _pear_ contains about 12% of the recommended dietary allowance for vitamin C, which is beneficial for protecting DNA, stopping cell mutation, maintaining a healthy metabolism and repairing tissue. _Pear_ is a high-fiber food which help lower cholesterol, sustain healthy blood sugar level and increase digestive health. Pears also contains a fair amount of vitamins K, B2, B3 and B6. As minerals, one pear contains calcium, magnesium, potassium, copper and manganese. It also contains folate for expecting or nursing mums.
Furthermore, it contains boron, which our bodies need in order to retain calcium, so this fruit can also be linked to prevention of osteoporosis. Quercetin is another antioxidant found in the skin of pears. It's beneficial for cancer prevention and can help reduce blood pressure, so don't peel your pears!

N.46   _Rice the Glory_   Yes / No

rice milk	½ cup
spinach	1 handful
mango	½
kiwi	2
dairy free rice pudding	½ cup
goji berry	1 tbsp

HOW TO: prepare the rice pudding in advance and let it cool down. Wash, peel and chop the fruits and the veggie and place it in the blender.

TIPS: To make rice pudding, first of all cook the rice in boiling water with a pinch of salt. Then combine in a saucepan the cooked rice, with a cup or more of rice milk and 1 tbsp of sugar. Stir until creamy.

ADD YOUR COMMENT: _____

_____

_____

N.47   _The Rich Pepper_   Yes / No

green pepper	½
red pepper	½
yellow pepper	½
avocado	1
spicy red paprika powder	½ tsp
turmeric	1 tsp
hemp milk	¾ cup

HOW TO: wash and chop all the veg and place it in the blender together with the other ingredients. Press START

TIPS: keep it 20 to 30 minutes in the fridge before to enjoy the blend.

ADD YOUR COMMENT: _____

_____

_____

N.48   *Gifts of Nature*   *Yes / No*

watercress	3 leaves
swiss chard	3 leaves
parsley	4 leaves
peach	2
almond milk	¾ cup
mix nuts	1 handful
lime zest	of 1 lime

HOW TO: wash and chop all the veg and fruits and place it in the blender. Grate the zest of one lime and add nuts and milk. Press START.

TIPS: there are so many milk options out there, pick the one you like the most.

ADD YOUR COMMENT: _____

_____

_____

N.49   *Dancing in the MoonLight*   *Yes / No*

kiwi	2
strawberry	6
kale	1 handful
carrot	3 large
ice	½ cup
maca powder	1 tsp
agave syrup	1 tsp

HOW TO: juice the carrots and place it in the blender with the ice, Maca powder and the syrup. Wash and chop the kale and add it to the mix. Peel and chop the kiwi and add it to the mix. Wash the strawberries and blend it together with the rest.

TIPS: I like to keep the top leafy part of the strawberry in the blender. But is a personal choice. With or without for you?

ADD YOUR COMMENT: _____

_____

_____

The chicky Drink   *Yes / No*

chickpeas	½ cup
cashew nuts	½ cup
avocado	½
almond milk	¾ cup

HOW TO: soak the cashew nuts in advance. Use the canned chickpeas or cook them yourself (it must be cold when you place it in the blender). Add all ingredients in the blender and press START

TIPS: add 1 tsp of maple syrup to balance the flavour

ADD YOUR COMMENT: _____

_____

_____

N.51   *The mango way*   *Yes / No*

green tea	¾ cup
mango	1
fruit of the forest	1 handful
lemon zest	of 1 lemon
chia seeds	1 tsp
fig	1

HOW TO: prepare the tea in advance. Zest one lemon and add the rest of the ingredients. Press START.

TIPS: I like to use frozen fruit of the forest so that my blend will stay fresh.

ADD YOUR COMMENT: _____

_____

_____

N.52 *The Zesty Flavour* *Yes / No*

liquorice	1 stick
coconut milk	¾ cup
banana	1
orange zest	of 1 whole orange
cantaloup melon	1 slice

HOW TO: wash and chop all the ingredients and place it in the blender. Press START.

TIPS: add more or less banana for a thicker or thinner smoothie

ADD YOUR COMMENT: _____

_____

_____

N.53 *The Almond Town* *Yes / No*

sweet potato	½
figs	3
almond butter	1 tbs
almond milk	¾ cup
flax seeds	1 tsp

HOW TO: in advance, boil a ½ sweet potato and let it cool down or run it under cold water. Place all the ingredients in the blender and press START

TIPS: most of the people don't eat the fig skin. I will say, take a fig, cut off the top and the bottom with the skin still on and then cut it in half to check the quality and place it in the blender. The skin gives extra thickness and extra flavour.

ADD YOUR COMMENT: _____

_____

_____

pineapple	⅓
turmeric	1 tbsp
black pepper (milled)	a pinch
ginger	20 ml
lime	1
orange	3
banana	1

HOW TO: juice the pineapple, orange and ginger. In the blender place the juice together with the banana, one squeezed lime, turmeric, ginger and a pinch of ground black pepper

TIPS: remove the central part of the pineapple…it taste real bitter!

ADD YOUR COMMENT: _____

_____

_____

THE W@W FACTOR: *Black Pepper* is the fruit of the black pepper plant from the *Piperaceae* family. Native to Kerala, the southern state of India, it is used as both, a spice and a medicine.

Black pepper is a rich source of minerals like manganese, copper, magnesium, calcium, phosphorus, iron, potassium, of vitamins like riboflavin, vitamin C, K, and B6 and has a high content of dietary fiber too.

In Ayurvedic practices, pepper is added to tonics for treating cold and cough. *Black Pepper* also provides relief from sinusitis and nasal congestion: it has an expectorant property that helps break up the mucus and phlegm depositions in the respiratory tract.

Piperine, one of the key components of black pepper, has been shown in numerous studies to reduce memory impairment and cognitive malfunction while providing an excellent depth of flavour to our dishes.

N.55   _The Leafy_   _Yes / No_

orange	3
radish	1
lettuce	3 leaves
banana	1 ½
celery	2 stalk
rocket	4 leaves

HOW TO: Juice only the oranges. Carefully wash and chop all the other ingredients and place it in the blender. Press START.

TIPS: play with the amount of rocket to give more or less strength to your blend.

ADD YOUR COMMENT: _____

_____

_____

N.56   _The Powder Power_   _Yes / No_

green tea	¾ cup
turmeric	1 tsp
maca	1 tsp
spirulina	1 tsp
avocado	½
banana	½
kale	1 handful

HOW TO: prepare the green tea by adding a little of hot water in a cup with the tea bag (use a tea spoon to force the flavour out) and fill the cup with cold water. Add all the ingredients in the blender and press START.

TIPS: if you are not a fun of green tea, use instead plain cold water with a couple of ice cubes.

ADD YOUR COMMENT: _____

_____

_____

N.57   _Be my own_   Yes / No

chia seeds	1 tsp
blueberries	1 handful
dairy free soy yoghurt	2 tbsp
acai berry	1 frozen cube
beetroot	½
ice	½ cup
banana	½

HOW TO: place all the ingredients in the blender and press START.

TIPS: acai can be found frozen or in powder. If you have the acai powder at home use 1 flat tbsp of measure in you blend.

ADD YOUR COMMENT: _____
_____
_____

N.58   _Fun the Night_   Yes / No

goji berry	1 tbsp
mix seeds	1 tbsp
dairy free plain ice cream	3 tbsp
blueberries	1 handful
maple syrup	1 tsp
banana	½
vanilla syrup	1 tsp
water	½ cup

HOW TO: you only need a blender! Mix all the ingredients and press START

TIPS: mix seeds: use a mix of linseed, chia seed, sesame seed, sunflower seeds and pumpkin seed.

ADD YOUR COMMENT: _____
_____
_____

The Sun is Up

muesli	2 tbsp
cocoa	1 tsp
banana	1
oat milk	¾ cup
strawberry	8

HOW TO: place all the ingredient in the blender and press START.

TIPS: instead of oat milk maybe try a vanilla soy milk for extra flavour

ADD YOUR COMMENT: _____

_____

_____

THE W@W FACTOR: *Strawberry* is a delicious seasonal hybrid species widely grown for the bright red colour, juice texture and sweetness of its fruit.

Strawberries are rich in antioxidant and nutrients including vitamin C, folate, potassium, manganese, dietary fiber and magnesium.

They are especially valuable for eye care: antioxidants such as flavonoids, phenolic phytochemicals, and ellagic acid, all of which are present in *strawberries*, can help avoid dry eyes, degeneration of the optic nerves, macular degeneration, vision defects, and increased susceptibility to infections. Also *strawberries* may help with the disturbance in ocular pressure. Any disturbance in this pressure can be harmful to the eyes. *Strawberries* are helpful because they contain potassium, which helps in maintaining the correct pressure.

Furthermore, strawberries are involved in improving heart health, promote skin care by acting as an anti-aging, reduce high blood pressure, prevent cancer, boost immunity, boosts brain function, reduce inflammation, help with constipation and diabetes.

coconut fat	1 tbsp
coconut flake	1 tbsp
strawberry	6
chocolate shaving	1 full tsp
coconut milk	¾ cup
banana	1
ice	5 cube

HOW TO: buy 1 can of fat coconut milk and keep it in the fridge overnight. Open the can in the morning and scoop the fat and place it in the blender. Add all the other ingredients and press START to smooth.

TIPS: if possible use dark chocolate shaving for a more intense flavour

ADD YOUR COMMENT: _____

_____

_____

One smoothie a day:
The juice section

This chapter has the aim to be blender free. You will discover 20 different juices idea for when you are only looking for a mid afternoon snack and want to avoid to feel too full. For this section is necessary the use of a juicer: don't wait any further! Shop for your juicer now and stop buying sugary juices in store.

Try all of them and cross one of the boxes on the side of each smoothie every time you find a blend that satisfy your palate in order to be able to come back to do only your favourites one.

Cross **Yes** if you like the smoothie

Cross **No** if you think is not for you

Plus, use the section ADD YOUR COMMENT to personalise your smoothie: if you like more apple or less basil, this is where you should jot down your thoughts and be the author of your life.

N.61   _Boost my body_   Yes / No

cucumber	½
celery	3 stalks
ginger	20 ml

HOW TO: wash all the vegetables and place them in the juicer.
TIPS: Shake it before to drink
ADD YOUR COMMENT: _____

_____

_____

N.62   A Wise Man   Yes / No

mandarin	1
carrot	1
spinach	1 handful
cucumber	⅓
honey dew melon	1 slice

HOW TO: wash carefully carrots, spinach and cucumber. Peel the mandarin and slice the melon. Juice your ingredients.
TIPS: leave it in the fridge for 20/30 minutes before to drink or add 2 ice cubes.
ADD YOUR COMMENT: _____

_____

_____

coconut water	½ cup
pineapple	1 slice
ice	3 cubes
carrot	1

HOW TO: chop in chunks the pineapple and carrot and juice them together. Add the coconut water and the ice cubes.

TIPS: if possible, keep the coconut water in the fridge for a couple of hours before to mix

ADD YOUR COMMENT: _____

_____

_____

THE W@W FACTOR: *carrot* is a root vegetable, usually orange in colour, probably originated in Persia. The most commonly eaten part of the plant is the taproot, although the stems and leaves are eaten as well.

Most of the benefits of the *carrots* comes from their beta-carotene and fiber content. They are also rich in vitamin A, C, K and B8, as well as pantothenic acid, folate, potassium, iron, copper and manganese.

They are a good source of antioxidants.

The health benefits of *carrots* include reduced cholesterol, lower risk of heart attack, cancer prevention, improve vision and fight sign of aging. Furthermore, improve digestion, detoxify the body and boost oral health.

N.64   _The Healthy Beat_   Yes / No

fennel	1
celery	1 stalk
carrot	2

HOW TO: wash all the ingredients, chop it and juice it.

TIPS: be the author of your smoothie, change the combination of element in order to satisfy your palate at best.

ADD YOUR COMMENT: _____

_____

_____

N.65   _Flame the Heal_   Yes / No

orange	1
peach	1
carrot	3
ginger	20 ml

HOW TO: wash and chop all of the ingredients and place them in the juicer

TIPS: always clean the juicer straight after the use. It's easier and healthier.

ADD YOUR COMMENT: _____

_____

_____

N.66   _Mix the taste_   Yes / No

carrot	2
kiwi	1
mango	1
spinach	1 handful

HOW TO: wash, chop and place all the ingredients in the juicer.

TIPS: sip as you go! There's no better taste that a juice just made.

ADD YOUR COMMENT: _____

_____

_____

N.67   _The Dark side of the Juice_   Yes / No

beetroot	2
apple	1
cucumber	⅓
celery	1 stalk

HOW TO: wash, chop and place all the ingredients in the juicer

TIPS: add a tsp of protein powder of your choice to turn it in a energizing drink

ADD YOUR COMMENT: _____

_____

_____

N.68   <u>Aloha~~~</u>   Yes / No

apple	1
pineapple	2 slices

HOW TO: place the ingredients in the juicer.

TIPS: cut out the central part of the pineapple; it's hard to blend and it's bitter.

ADD YOUR COMMENT: _____

_____

_____

N.69   <u>It grows on me</u>   Yes / No

kale	1 handful
grapes	~20
carrot	3 large

HOW TO: wash, chop and place all the ingredients in the juicer

TIPS: you don't need to peel the carrots for a juicer. The machine will do the job for you. You may need to chop the carrots depends on the size of the juicer.

ADD YOUR COMMENT: _____

_____

_____

N.70   _Sweat Away_   Yes / No

green tea	½ cup
watermelon	1 slice
spirulina powder	1 tsp

HOW TO: juice the watermelon. Add the green tea. Add 1 tsp of spirulina and stir.

TIPS: why don't you freeze your juice and eat it like a sorbet? this is a lovely idea to involve your little one in the juice making process

ADD YOUR COMMENT: _____
_____
_____

N.71   _Light in life_   Yes / No

kiwi	1
mango	½
pineapple	1 slice
strawberry	4
blueberry	7

HOW TO: wash carefully all of the ingredients. Juice them all!

TIPS: remember, your juice can also be a sorbet. Have fun with it and show it off with your friends.

ADD YOUR COMMENT: _____
_____
_____

N.72   *Bloody Good*   *Yes / No*

carrot	2
beetroot	1
celery	1 stick

HOW TO: wash and chop all the veg and place it in the juicer

TIPS: add little agave syrup to sweeten the taste if you find it necessary

ADD YOUR COMMENT: _____

_____

_____

N.73   *Cleanse me up*   *Yes / No*

pineapple	1 slice
green tea	½ cup
spinach	1 handful

HOW TO: prepare the tea in advance. Juice the pineapple and the spinach. Add the tea to the juice

TIPS: remember to cut the central part of the pineapple before to juice it.

ADD YOUR COMMENT: _____

_____

_____

grapefruit	1
carrot	2
apple	1
strawberry	4
grapes	5

HOW TO: wash thoroughly all your fruits and vegetables before to juice it.

TIPS: Play with the amount of grapefruit to add to your juice in order to gain a more or less bitter flavoured juice. Also if you like have extra freshness try to add few mint leaves to the mix.

ADD YOUR COMMENT: _____

_____

_____

THE W@W FACTOR: *grapefruit* is a subtropical citrus tree known for its sour to semi-sweet fruit. *Grapefruit* is a hybrid originating in Barbados as an accidental cross between two introduced species, sweet orange and pomelo. The fruit is yellow-orange skinned and generally has a spheroid shape. The name *grapefruit* was given because of it tendency to grow in clusters, like grapes.

When it come to it nutritional value, grapefruit contains plenty of vitamin C, vitamin A, calcium, magnesium, vitamin E, thiamine, riboflavin, niacin, folate, pantothenic acid, potassium, phosphorus, manganese, zinc, and copper. It also contains lycopene, beta-carotene and active plant compound that turn the grapefruit in a powerful antioxidant for the body helping to fight skin damage, reduce wrinkles and improve overall skin texture.

Grapefruit is also very good to boost the immune system against cold and other common illness, reduce fatigue, treat indigestion, promote sleep, reduce acidity, eliminate constipation, remove flatulence, treat urinary disorders, reduce risk of diabetes and heart conditions.

Furthermore, the high amount of fiber in these fruit helps release cholecystokinin in the body, a hormone that acts as a natural hunger suppressant, helping people avoid overeating and making them feel sated.

N.75   _The Super Juice_   Yes / No

apple	½
carrot	1
fennel	½
cucumber	⅓
beetroot	½
spirulina	1 tsp

HOW TO: wash, chop and juice all the ingredients. Mix one tsp of spirulina powder to the juice. Stir well!

TIPS: feel free to change the powder with any other you may have already available in your cupboard

ADD YOUR COMMENT: _____

_____

_____

N.76   _One with the Ground_   Yes / No

lettuce	3 large leaves
spinach	1 handful
apple	1 and ½
pear	2
kale	1 handful

HOW TO: wash, chop and juice all the ingredients

TIPS: add ice cubes for freshness

ADD YOUR COMMENT: _____

_____

_____

N.77   *Land of Grow*   *Yes / No*

    cucumber   ¾
    celery   3 stalks

HOW TO: wash and juice the ingredients.

TIPS: add maple syrup if you need to

ADD YOUR COMMENT: _____
_____
_____

N.78   *A better Skin*   *Yes / No*

    green tea   ½ cup
    kale   1 handful
    mango   1

HOW TO: prepare the green tea in advance. Juice the kale and the mango and mix it with the tea

TIPS: let it rest in the fridge for 30 minutes before to drink it.

ADD YOUR COMMENT: _____
_____
_____

N.79 _Nurturing Way_ Yes / No

orange	1
mango	1
ginger	20 ml
ice	4 cubes

HOW TO: wash, peel and juice all the ingredients. Add the ice in the end, straight in the glass.

TIPS: drink one juice/smoothie every day to reduce heaviness on your stomach

ADD YOUR COMMENT: _____

_____

_____

N.80 _Simplicity_ Yes / No

apple	1 ½
orange	1 ½

HOW TO: wash and chop the apples. Wash and peel the oranges. Juice it all!

TIPS: often, the easiest the juice the tastier!

ADD YOUR COMMENT: _____

_____

_____

One smoothie a day:
The Baby Love

This chapter gift you with 20 incredibly tasty smoothie bowl recipes that are loved from the little one of every age. Don't miss out! Share this full of flavour smoothies' alternative with your little one… or enjoy for yourself this perfectly balanced blend of goodness.

Namaste

Try all of them and cross one of the boxes on the side of each smoothie every time you find a blend that satisfy your palate in order to be able to come back to do only your favourites one.

Cross **Yes** if you like the smoothie

Cross **No** if you think is not for you

Plus, use the section ADD YOUR COMMENT to personalise your smoothie: if you like more apple or less basil, this is where you should jot down your thoughts and be the author of your life.

N.81   <u>*The Kids Friendly Drink*</u>   *Yes / No*

banana	1 and ½
strawberry	7
apple	2

HOW TO: wash thoroughly all the fruits. Peel the bananas and take the green part of the strawberries away. Blend it all

TIPS: place it in a bowl and allow your kid to scoop his way through it

ADD YOUR COMMENT: _____

_____

_____

N.82   *The Kids Breakfast*   *Yes / No*

blueberry	1 handful
dairy free blueberry yoghurt	4 scoops
banana	1
kiwi	3
oats	1 tbsp

HOW TO: juice only the kiwis. Blend all the other ingredients with the kiwi juice as base.

TIPS: add water if you need more liquids base

ADD YOUR COMMENT: _____

_____

_____

N.83   *The Kids Cookie meal*   *Yes / No*

vegan friendly cookie	2
almond yoghurt	5 tbsp
oats	1 tbsp
cocoa	1 tbsp
water	½ cup

HOW TO: place all the ingredients in the blender and press START

TIPS: place it in a smoothie bowl and and enjoy it

ADD YOUR COMMENT: _____

_____

_____

N.84   _Fruit Up_   Yes / No

plums	2
carrot juiced and chunked	3
peach	2
ice	5

HOW TO: juice 2 carrots and boil the third until soft (if you have a high speed blender you can simply chop the carrot and let the blender do the job for you!). Chop the soft boiled carrot and place it in the blender together with all the other ingredients. Press START.

TIPS: scoop your smoothie

ADD YOUR COMMENT: _____

_____

_____

N.85   _Cookie Love_   Yes / No

vegan friendly cookies	2
strawberry	6
cocoa	1 tbsp
almond milk	1 cup

HOW TO: wash the strawberries and place all the ingredients in your blender. Press START.

TIPS: perfect for a kids play date

ADD YOUR COMMENT: _____

_____

_____

N.86   _Happy Tummy_   Yes / No

banana	2
mango	2
agave syrup	2 tsp
ice	4 cubes

HOW TO: juice the mangoes and blend it with the banana and the ice. Add the syrup only if you feel the need of extra sweetness in your bowl.

TIPS: you can avoid ice by adding ⅓ cup of cold spring water.

ADD YOUR COMMENT: _____

_____

_____

N.87   _Strawberries' heart_   Yes / No

kiwi	2
carrot	2
banana	1
strawberries	10

HOW TO: juice the carrots and place it together with the other ingredients in the blender. Press START.

TIPS: add water if you need bigger quantity or have it more juicy

ADD YOUR COMMENT: _____

_____

_____

N.88 _Peach a Dream_ *Yes / No*

peach	4
dairy free plain yoghurt	2 tbsp
banana	1
water	½ cup
ice	2 cubes

HOW TO: place all the ingredients in the blender and press START.

TIPS: remember to take out the stone from the peaches.

ADD YOUR COMMENT: _____

_____

_____

N.89 _I've been Good_   *Yes / No*

dairy free chocolate ice cream	2 tbsp
soy milk	½ cup
banana	1
chocolate chips	1 tbsp
ice	4 cubes

HOW TO: place all the ingredients in the blender and press START

TIPS: place the smoothie in a bowl and add extra chocolate chips on top. It will be gone before you even notice it.

ADD YOUR COMMENT: _____

_____

_____

N.90   _Sweet Tooth_   *Yes / No*

dairy free vanilla ice cream	2 tbsp
strawberries	6
vanilla soy milk	½ cup
ice	2 cubes
banana	1
cinnamon	1 tsp

HOW TO: place all the ingredients in the blender and press START

TIPS: remind your kid how much you love him by sharing this gorgeous and tasty meal.

ADD YOUR COMMENT: _____

_____

_____

N.91   _Fresh on Earth_   *Yes / No*

apple	2
strawberry	6
blueberry	1 handful
mint	3 leaves

HOW TO: place all the ingredients in the blender and press START

TIPS: for your kid is better remove the green top part of the strawberry. They may not enjoying the peculiar taste

ADD YOUR COMMENT: _____

_____

_____

N.92   _The Rich Meal_   *Yes / No*

granola	2 tbsp
kiwi	1
fig	2
coconut yoghurt	3 spoons
coconut milk	½ cup
avocado	½
cocoa	1 tbsp

HOW TO: place all the ingredients in the blender and press START

TIPS: this is a highly nutritional meal. Good for a lunch alternative!

ADD YOUR COMMENT: _____
_____
_____

N.93   _Nutty Taste_   *Yes / No*

mix nuts	2 tbsp
almond milk	¾ cup
almond butter	2 tbsp
banana	1

HOW TO: place all the ingredients in the blender and press START

TIPS: be careful with the nuts! Make sure they are well grounded and that there are not stones or sharp edges mix in between.

ADD YOUR COMMENT: _____
_____
_____

N.94   *Little Baby Grow*   *Yes / No*

green tea	1 cup
pear	3 small
peach	3

HOW TO: prepare the tea in advance and let it cool down. Add all the ingredients in the blender and press START

TIPS: if your little one doesn't find it sweet enough you may always add some agave syrup.

ADD YOUR COMMENT: _____

_____

_____

N.95   *Friends Attraction*   *Yes / No*

dairy free chocolate ice cream	3 tbsp
strawberries	5
blueberries	1 handful
avocado	½
chocolate soy milk	1 cup
agave syrup	1 tsp

HOW TO: blend all the ingredients together

TIPS: be the envy of all the other mum with this highly nutritional, yet super yummy smoothie/smoothie bowl

ADD YOUR COMMENT: _____

_____

_____

N.96   *The Young Exotic*   Yes / No

coconut water	½ cup
pineapple	1 slice
watermelon	1 slice

HOW TO: place all the ingredients in the blender and press START

TIPS: is ideal in hot sunny day to refresh the it body.

ADD YOUR COMMENT: _____

_____

_____

N.97   *Drink your Snack*   Yes / No

kiwi	2
fig	2
ice	½ cup
mint	3 leaves
avocado	½
banana	½

HOW TO: blend all the ingredients together

TIPS: if you like it more juicy, add ⅓ cup of water or fresh apple juice

ADD YOUR COMMENT: _____

_____

_____

N.98   *It's that Good?*   Yes / No

chocolate chip	1 tbsp
raspberry	1 handful
date	2
hemp milk	¾ cup

HOW TO: place all the ingredients in the mixer to blend

TIPS: pour it in your smoothie bowl and top it with few raspberries and chocolate chips

ADD YOUR COMMENT: _____

_____

_____

N.99   *Grapes Fun*   Yes / No

blueberries	1 handful
yellow grapes	15
soy milk	½ cup
kale	1 handful

HOW TO: blend all the ingredients together

TIPS: add cinnamon for extra flavour

ADD YOUR COMMENT: _____

_____

_____

N.100   *Kids Love*   *Yes / No*

apple	2
mango	1
kiwi	1
spinach	1 handful

HOW TO: simply blend all together

TIPS: can be drink any time anywhere
       Don't be shy!

ADD YOUR COMMENT: _____

_____

_____

One smoothie a day:
The Guilty Pleasure

This chapter is gifted with some naughty ideas to share on a friends night or to keep for your secret moments. Soon, you are going to discover 10 different recipes containing alcohol mix with that fruits and vegetables that we love so much.

Life is all about balance!!!

Enjoy this guilty pleasure

Try all of them and cross one of the boxes on the side of each smoothie every time you find a blend that satisfy your palate in order to be able to come back to do only your favourites one.

Cross *Yes* if you like the smoothie

Cross *No* if you think is not for you

Plus, use the section ADD YOUR COMMENT to personalise your smoothie: if you like more apple or less basil, this is where you should jot down your thoughts and be the author of your life.

N.101   *The exotic Spice*   *Yes / No*

pineapple	½
cherry	8
passion fruit	1
vodka	30 ml
turmeric	1 tsp

HOW TO: juice the pineapple. Blend the pineapple juice together with the pitted cherry, scooped passion fruit and turmeric. Add the vodka in the end and stir.

TIPS: place it in a fancy glass and add an extra cherry for decoration.

ADD YOUR COMMENT: _____
_____
_____

N.102   *Sexy plus*   *Yes / No*

soaked cashew nuts   ½ cup
cherry   1 handful
almond milk   ½ cup
amarena cherry syrup   1 tbsp
gin   25 ml
raspberry   1 handful
lime squeeze   ½ lime

HOW TO: soak the cashew nuts in advance. Blend all the ingredients together

TIPS: pour it in a cocktail glass and top with some more amarena cherry syrup

ADD YOUR COMMENT: _____
_____
_____

N.103   *The Guilty Dinner*   *Yes / No*

whisky   25ml
olives   10
water   1 cup
oregano   a pinch
tomato   1 large
salt   a pinch
potato   1 small

HOW TO: boil the potato in advance and let it cool down. Mix all the other ingredients in the blender and press START

TIPS: pour it in a cocktail glass and use as decoration a toothpick with 2 olives…..preferably green olives.

ADD YOUR COMMENT: _____
_____
_____

N.104   _The Hungarian_   _Yes / No_

palinka	25 ml
apricot	1
pear	1
plum 1	
sweet yellow paprika	1
cherry	3
yellow grapes	5
ice	½ cup

HOW TO: blend all the ingredients together

TIPS: pour it in a cocktail glass and decorate it with a toothpick with a cherry and a piece of plum.

ADD YOUR COMMENT: _____

_____

_____

N.105   _The Guilty Pleasure_   _Yes / No_

vodka	25 ml
apple	1
strawberry	5
blueberry	1 handful
chocolate chip	1 tbsp
ice	½ cup
maple syrup	1 tsp
optional (soy whipped cream on top)	
chocolate syrup to top	

HOW TO: juice the apple and then blend all the ingredients together.

TIPS: pour it in a cocktail glass and top with some soy whipped cream, chocolate syrup and chocolate chip

ADD YOUR COMMENT: _____

_____

_____

N.106   _The Guilty Vegetables_   Yes / No

parsley	4 leaves
apricot	1
cucumber	1
vodka	25 ml
spinach	1 handful
avocado	½
pear	1 small
ice	4 cubes
agave syrup to garnish the glass	

HOW TO: juice the cucumber and then blend all the ingredients together

TIPS: pour the smoothie in a cocktail glass and garnish with agave syrup

ADD YOUR COMMENT: _____

_____

_____

N.107   _The Guilty Summer_   Yes / No

watermelon	1 slice
gin	20 ml
vodka	20 ml
passion fruit	1
papaya	1
mango	½
mango syrup to garnish	

HOW TO: juice the watermelon. Blend all the other ingredients together

TIPS: pour the blend in a cocktail glass and garnish with mango syrup

ADD YOUR COMMENT: _____

_____

_____

N.108   *The Guilty Autumn*   *Yes / No*

raisin	1 handful
rum	25 ml
dairy free vanilla ice cream	3 tbsp
cinnamon	1 tsp
banana	1
ice	½ cup

HOW TO: blend all the ingredients together

TIPS: pour it in a cocktail glass and garnish with agave syrup

ADD YOUR COMMENT: _____

_____

_____

N.109   *The Guilty and more*   *Yes / No*

sparkling water	½ cup
gin	25 ml
banana	1
papaya	1 small
cantaloupe melon	1 slice
passion fruit syrup to decorate	

HOW TO: blend all the ingredients together

TIPS: pour it in a cocktail glass and garnish with passion fruit syrup. Leave also some passion fruit seed on the bottom for a better look.

ADD YOUR COMMENT: _____

_____

_____

N.110   <u>*The Guilty Whisky*</u>   *Yes / No*

whisky	25 ml
plum	1
coriander	3 leaves
kiwi	1
cucumber	1

HOW TO: juice the cucumber and mix all the ingredients in the blender. Press START

TIPS: garnish with a slice of cucumber

ADD YOUR COMMENT: _____

_____

_____

One smoothie a day:
All the way to the end

This chapter represent the most comprehensive part of the book with 220 smoothie recipes to accompany you for most of this year seasons. You will find several W@W factor to help you understand how smoothies can help your metabolism. You will also be able to experience unusual combinations of items and get to try very exotic fruits and vegetables.

I will type on the side of each smoothie's name if it is better to be consume over breakfast, lunch/dinner or as dessert in order to help you find your ideal smoothie whenever you are looking for it

Get ready with your juicer and blender, clear your shelf and have fun shopping.

We are getting serious!

P.s. Try one new every day an observe your skin changing before your eyes.

Try all of them and cross one of the boxes on the side of each smoothie every time you find a blend that satisfy your palate in order to be able to come back to do only your favourites one.

Cross **Yes** if you like the smoothie

Cross **No** if you think is not for you

Plus, use the section ADD YOUR COMMENT to personalise your smoothie: if you like more apple or less basil, this is where you should jot down your thoughts and be the author of your life.

N.111	_Aloe Supreme_	Yes / No
	#lunch/dinner	

avocado	½
kiwi	2
fig	3
aloe vera	½ cup
peanut butter	1 tbsp

HOW TO: wash and chop all the ingredients and blend.

TIPS: Peel only the avocado and the kiwi. No need to peel the skin out of the fig. You can simply chop the top and the bottom of the fig and place it in the blender.

ADD YOUR COMMENT: _____
_____
_____

N.112   _The seed art_   Yes / No
#lunch/dinner

hemp seed	1 tsp
chia seed	1 tsp
flaxseed	1 tsp
pumpkin seed	1 tsp
almonds	1 tbsp
avocado	1
mint	5 leaves
apple	2 ½

HOW TO: juice only the apples and then blend everything together.

TIPS: create a smoothie bowl with this blend and add more seeds on top for decoration.

ADD YOUR COMMENT: _____
_____
_____

N.113   _The Wind of the East_   Yes / No
#breakfast /lunch/dinner

rice pudding	½ cup
dates	3
frozen berry	1 handful
lime	½
apple	2

HOW TO: prepare the rice pudding in advance. Juice the apples and lime. Blend all the ingredients together.

TIPS: if you like, you can already cook the dates together with the pudding to make it moister and with a unique texture.

ADD YOUR COMMENT: _____
_____
_____

Mint in Action

#lunch/dinner

cucumber	½
carrot	2 whole
avocado	1
mint	~15 leaves

HOW TO: juice the cucumber and the carrots and then place it in the blender together with the avocado and mint

TIPS: add a pinch of spirulina powder for extra strength

ADD YOUR COMMENT: _____
_____
_____

THE W@W FACTOR: The mentha, or *mint*, family refers to a group of around 13 to 18 plant species, including peppermint and spearmint.

Mint is a calming and soothing herb that has been used for thousands of years to aid with upset stomach or indigestion: it has one of the highest antioxidant capacities of any food.

Mint is great to fight common cold because it contains menthol which is a natural aromatic decongestant that helps to break up phlegm and mucus, making it easier to expel. Also menthol has a cooling effect and can help relieve a sore throat.
And lets not forget that *mint* is a natural breath freshener.

When it comes to nutritional value mint contains small amount of potassium, magnesium, calcium, phosphorus, iron, vitamin C and vitamin A.

The Cocobanana

#breakfast

coconut yoghurt	½ cup
coconut milk	¾ cup
banana	1
berry (mix frozen)	1 handful
kiwi	1

HOW TO: place all the ingredient in a blender and press START

TIPS: plain soy yoghurt could be a valid alternative to coconut yoghurt should you don't have it available to your nearest grocery store. Don't forget to peel the kiwi before to place it in the blender.

ADD YOUR COMMENT: _____

_____

_____

THE W@W FACTOR: The *Coconut* tree is a member of the palm family. It is high in ascorbic acid, vitamin B, proteins, calcium, potassium and magnesium. The water in the *coconut* is one of the highest sources of electrolytes which are responsible for keeping the body properly hydrated so the muscles and nerves can function appropriately.

Coconut water is also low in calories, carbohydrates, and sugars, and almost completely fat-free.

Eating *coconuts* also supports the development of strong, healthy bones and teeth by improving the body's ability to absorb calcium and magnesium. It helps keep hair and skin healthy, prevents wrinkles, sagging skin, age spots, and provides sun protection.

Coconut oil is high in natural saturated fats which not only increase the healthy cholesterol in our body, but also help convert the bad cholesterol into good cholesterols. The increased good cholesterol helps then promote heart health and lower the risk of heart disease.

Popeye's choice   Yes / No

#snack/dinner

| apple | 3 whole |
| spinach | 2 handful |

HOW TO: juice the apples. Pour the juice in the blender. Add your spinach and press START.

TIPS: don't forget to wash your fruit and vegetable properly before to start.

ADD YOUR COMMENT: _____

_____

_____

THE W@W FACTOR: *Spinach* is an edible flowering plant native to central and western Asia. Low in fat and even lower in cholesterol, spinach is high in niacin and zinc, as well as protein, fiber, vitamins A, C, E and K, thiamin, vitamin B6, folate, calcium, iron, magnesium, phosphorus, potassium, copper, and manganese.

The possible health benefits of consuming spinach are many and include improving blood glucose control in people with diabetes, lowering the risk of cancer, reducing blood pressure, improving bone health, lowering the risk of developing asthma, prevent constipation and promote a healthy digestive tract.

Also, an adequate intake of iron-rich food like spinach helps prevent hair loss, commonly caused by iron deficiency.

Furthermore, spinach is high in vitamin A, which is necessary for sebum production to keep hair moisturized.

Vitamin A is also necessary for the growth of all bodily tissues, including skin and hair.

I have a date   *Yes / No*

#breakfast

soaked cashew nuts	½ cup
dates	4 cup
almond milk	¾ cup

HOW TO: soak the cashew nuts overnight or bring it to boil for twenty minutes. Add all the ingredients to the blender and press START

TIPS: make sure to pit the dates before to place them in the blender.

ADD YOUR COMMENT: _____

_____

_____

THE W@W FACTOR: *Date* is a flowering plant belonging to the palm family cultivated for its edible sweet fruit. Although its place of origin is unknown, it probably originated from the area between Egypt and Mesopotamia.

Dates contain a wide range of vitamins such as B1, B2, B3 and B5, as well as A1 and C: eat one *date* a day and no more vitamin supplements needed. Plus, there will be a noticeable change in your energy levels.

Dates are also rich in selenium, manganese, copper, and magnesium, and all of these are required when it comes to keeping our bones healthy, and preventing conditions such as osteoporosis.

Did you know that *dates* are free from cholesterol, and contain very little fat? Including them in smaller quantities in your daily diet can help you keep a check on cholesterol level, and even assist in weight loss.

N.118   _Ground the Flow_   Yes / No
#dinner

mandarin	2
dates	2
peanut butter	1 tbsp
ginger	15 ml
mango	1
wheatgrass powder	1 tsp
romaine lettuce	5 leaves
ice	6 cubes

HOW TO: juice the mandarin, ginger, mango and lettuce. Blend the juice with the other ingredients.

TIPS: Add more ginger for a deep, intense cleanse

ADD YOUR COMMENT: _____
_____
_____

The Naughty Health Yes / No
#breakfast

chocolate shaving	1 tbsp
cocoa	1 tbsp
maca powder	1 tsp
green tea	¾ cup
banana	1
avocado	½
mint	4 leaves
ice	3 cubes

HOW TO: prepare the green tea in advance and then blend everything together.

TIPS: if you don't want to use a green tea bag, you have the option to mix 1 tsp of maca powder with plain water.

ADD YOUR COMMENT: _____

_____

_____

N.120   _Spin_   Yes / No

#breakfast

almond shaves	1 tbsp
coconut water	¾ cup
banana	1 ½
spirulina	1 tsp

HOW TO: blend all the ingredients together

TIPS: keep it in the fridge for half an hour before to drink

ADD YOUR COMMENT: _____

_____

_____

N.121   _Never give up_   Yes / No

#dessert

beetroot	1
dairy free vanilla Ice cream	2 tbsp
cucumber	½
fig	2
ice	½ cup

HOW TO: juice the cucumber and the beetroot and blend it with the rest.

TIPS: leave the skin of the figs on when blending, take off only the tip and the bottom.

ADD YOUR COMMENT: _____

_____

_____

N.122   *Countryside Love*   Yes / No

#lunch

aubergine	⅓
zucchini	½
potato	1 small
salt	a pinch
cucumber	½
celery	3 stalks
pear	1
ice	4 cubes

HOW TO: cook in advance aubergine, zucchini and potato with a bit if salt in boiling water. When tender allow them to cool down. Juice the cucumber and celery. Blend all together.

TIPS: Add little agave syrup for a more interesting flavour.

ADD YOUR COMMENT: _____

_____

_____

N.123   *Zesty green*   Yes / No

#lunch/dinner

kale	1 handful
avocado	½
lime zest	of 1 lime
pineapple	1 cup of juice
mango cubes ½	

HOW TO: juice the pineapple. Place the other ingredients in the blender and press START

TIPS: while slicing the pineapple, cut out the central part. It's hard to juice and is of a more bitter flavour

ADD YOUR COMMENT: _____

_____

_____

The Berry +++

#breakfast/lunch

goji berry	1 tbsp
strawberry	~ 4
blueberry	1 tbsp
raspberry	1 tbsp
blackberry	1 tbsp
cranberry	1 tbsp
cherry	~ 4
acai berry	(powder 1 tsp or frozen 1 piece)
soy yoghurt	¾ cup
ice	3 cubes

HOW TO: place all the ingredients in the blender and press START

TIPS: make sure the cherries are pitted

ADD YOUR COMMENT: _____

_____

_____

THE W@W FACTOR: *Goji berry* or 'wolfberry' is the fruit of a plant, native to Asia, belonging to the nightshade family. The same family that also includes potato, tomato, eggplant, belladonna, chili pepper, and tobacco. It contains vitamins A, C, B2, selenium, potassium, iron, calcium, fiber, proteins, amino acids, phytochemicals including beta-carotene and many more. Like most other superfoods, *goji berries* are an excellent source of antioxidants that help boost the immune system and protect the body from high levels of inflammation since they fight free radical damage.

*Goji berrie*s are loaded with beta-carotene, which helps promote healthy skin and even acts like a natural skin cancer treatment. Its benefits also include the ability to protect eyes from age-related diseases like macular degeneration, because of their high levels of antioxidants (especially zeaxanthin), which can help stop damage from UV light exposure, free radicals and other forms of oxidative stress.

Especially useful for people with diabetes by helping control the release of sugar into the bloodstream.

Traditionally, the Chinese call *Goji* the Matrimony Vine and believe them to have a big effect on the reproductive system and improving fertility by increasing the sperm count and the vitality of sperm and by treating female infertility in patients with premature ovarian failure and the inability to ovulate normally.

N.125   *Extraterrestrial Bomb*   *Yes / No*
          #lunch

papaya	1
mango	½
watermelon	2 slices (~¾ cup)
kale	1 handful
ginger	15 ml
wasabi	½ sachet (around 15 gr)
banana	½

HOW TO: juice only the watermelon. Mix all the other ingredients and blend.

TIPS: be careful! Is a very spicy smoothie, which makes it great if you have a block nose or sore throat but definitely not advice if you are not use to have spice in your diet.

ADD YOUR COMMENT: _____

_____

_____

N.126   *A clean Liver*   Yes / No
#dinner

celery	5 stalk
lime	½
avocado	1
mint	3 leaves
ice	½ cup
maple syrup (optional)	

HOW TO: juice celery and lime. Blend all the ingredients together.

TIPS: add the maple syrup only if you feel that the flavour is too strong for you.

ADD YOUR COMMENT: _____

_____

_____

The Grow that Blow   *Yes / No*

#lunch/dinner

tomatoes	1 whole
spinach	1 handful
cucumber	1 whole
celery	2 stalk
red bell pepper	½

HOW TO: juice only cucumber and celery and then add all the ingredients into the blender and press START

TIPS: add a wheatgrass powder for a energy boost. If you like a more juicy mix you can actually juice all of the ingredients above (you will be amazed by how much juice comes out from a pepper, a tomato or a bunch of spinach). Do you want to go juice free? Then chop ½ cucumber and 1 celery stalk into the blender and add either ½ cup of ice or plain water

ADD YOUR COMMENT: _____

_____

_____

THE W@W FACTOR: *Tomatoes* originated from the Andes, in what is now called Peru, Bolivia, Chile and Ecuador - where they grew wild. They were first cultivated by the Aztecs and Incas as early as 700 AD. Considered nowadays either a fruit that a vegetable they hold a wealth of nutrients and vitamins within, including an impressive amount of vitamin A, vitamin C, and vitamin K, as well as significant amounts of vitamin B6, folate, and thiamine.

They are also a good source of potassium, manganese, magnesium, phosphorus, and copper. Plus they have dietary fiber and protein that contribute to their health benefits.

The health benefits of *tomatoes* include eye care, good stomach health and a reduced blood pressure. They provide relief from diabetes, skin problems, and urinary tract infections. Furthermore, they improve digestion, stimulate blood circulation, reduce cholesterol levels, improve fluid balance, protect the kidneys, detoxify the body, prevent premature aging, and reduce inflammation.

N.128   *The Iron Plus*   Yes / No

#lunch

beetroot	2
spinach	1 handful
kale	1 handful
parsley	6 leaves
carrot	4
ice	4 cubes
avocado	½
maple syrup	1 tsp

HOW TO: juice carrots and beetroot. Add all the other ingredients to the blender and press START

TIPS: the secret ingredient is the parsley. See if your friends can guess this detail.

ADD YOUR COMMENT: _____

_____

_____

N.129   _Obscure Secret_   Yes / No
#lunch/dinner

black beans	2 tbsp
beetroot	2
carrot	2
pear	2
lemon zest	of 1 lemon
ice	½ cup

HOW TO: juice the carrots and beetroot. Blend it all!

TIPS: use pre-cooked beans from the can. It makes your blend faster.

ADD YOUR COMMENT: _____
_____
_____

Earth Paradise   _Yes / No_

#lunch

pumpkin puree (canned or fresh)	1 tbsp
cucumber	1 ½
turmeric (powder or grated)	1 tsp
red paprika powder	½ tsp
green bell pepper	1
mango	1

HOW TO: juice only the cucumber, add all the other ingredients to the blender and press START

TIPS: add a little maple syrup to the blend if you like to sweeter the taste

ADD YOUR COMMENT: _____

_____

_____

THE W@W FACTOR: _Mangoes_ are juicy stone fruit originated in southern Asia, almost 4,000 years ago. _Mango's_ cultivation first spread to Malaysia, eastern Asia, and eastern Africa and was finally introduced to California in the nineteenth century. According to Indian beliefs, _mangoes_ symbolize life and are used in many sacred ritual.

Mangoes are very low in saturated fat, cholesterol, and sodium. They are an excellent source of dietary fiber and vitamin B6, vitamin A, vitamin C, vitamin E, and vitamin K which help enhance the immune system and delay the ageing process.

They are also rich in minerals like potassium, magnesium, and copper, and they are one of the best sources of quercetin, beta-carotene, and astragalin. These powerful antioxidants help to neutralize free radicals throughout the body which means to prevent heart diseases, premature ageing, cancer, and degenerative diseases which are all due to these free radicals that damage the cells. They also contain selenium, calcium, iron, and phosphorus.

Mangoes are rich in iron, which makes them beneficial for people suffering from anemia by increasing the red blood cell count in the body. Because of its high iron content is also very much advised during pregnancy.

N.131   _Fury Coconut_   Yes / No

#lunch

spinach	1 handful
broccoli	⅓
celery	1 stalk
banana	½
coconut milk	½ cup
ground coconut	1 tbsp
coconut cream	1 tbsp
turmeric	1 tsp

HOW TO: blend all the ingredients together

TIPS: extract the coconut cream from the coconut milk can. Keep the can in the fridge overnight to naturally separate the fat from the liquid.

ADD YOUR COMMENT: _____

_____

_____

N.132   _Chunky Funk_   Yes / No

#lunch/dinner

carrot chunk	1
apple chunk	1
ice cubes	½ cup
ginger zest	10 gr or 1 tsp

HOW TO: boil slightly the carrots in order to make it tender. Blend all together.

TIPS: add water for a less thick compost

ADD YOUR COMMENT: _____

_____

_____

The Pumpkin Head

#lunch

banana	½
pumpkin puree	2 tbsp
avocado	½
maple syrup	1 tbsp
dairy free yoghurt	2 tbsp
apple	2 ½
ice cube	3 cubes

HOW TO: juice the apples and add all the other ingredients to the blender and press the START button

TIPS: add one tsp of spirulina powder to make this mix even more energising

ADD YOUR COMMENT: _____
_____
_____

THE W@W FACTOR: *Pumpkin* is a squash plant, round in shape, with smooth, slightly ribbed skin, and deep yellow to orange coloration.

Native to North America, *pumpkins* are mainly popular has a decoration during Halloween and as main ingredient in the delicious pumpkin pie.
It's a great source of potassium and beta-carotene.

It also contains some minerals including calcium and magnesium, as well as vitamins E, vitamin C and some B vitamins.

Its main health benefit is the big impact on maintaining a healthy skin: it helps with wound healing, to protect against sun damage and prevent dryness of the skin.

N.134   _The Dragon Rice_   Yes / No

#lunch

rice pudding	½ cup
dragon fruit	¾
mango	½
kale	1 handful
oat milk	½ cup
spirulina	1 tsp

HOW TO: prepare the rice pudding in advance. Blend all the ingredients together

TIPS: keep the blend in the fridge for 30 minutes before to drink

ADD YOUR COMMENT: _____

_____ _____

_____

N.135   _Jelly Freshness_   Yes / No

#lunch/dinner

aloe vera	1 cup
apricot	1
peach	1
swiss chart	1 handful
ice	6 cubes

HOW TO: blend all the ingredients together

TIPS: add some wheatgrass powder for extra boost

ADD YOUR COMMENT: _____

_____

_____

Spice Up the Night

Yes / No

#breakfast/lunch/dinner

passion fruit	1
orange	1
cantaloupe melon	2 slices
mint	5-6 leaves
ginger	25ml

HOW TO: juice the orange, the melon slices and the ginger. Scoop the passion fruit pulp and add it to the blender together with the mint and the juiced ingredients.

TIPS: juice and blend fruit and vegetable may tend to hit them. Avoid drink a warm mix by adding ice cubes to the blend or use frozen fruit.

ADD YOUR COMMENT: _____

_____

_____

THE W@W FACTOR: *Passion fruit* are round or oval fruit that can be yellow, red, purple or green in colour and have a juice edible centre composed of numerous seeds.

Passion fruit have a high number of nutrients which includes antioxidants, flavonoids, vitamin A, vitamin C, riboflavin, niacin, iron, magnesium, phosphorus, potassium, copper, fiber and protein.

All those nutrients allow for a wide range of benefits that goes from enhance digestion, prevent cancerous grow, improve eyesight, increase skin health, lower blood pressure, regulate fluid exchange in the body and improve bone mineral density. Furthermore, helps in the treatment of many respiratory conditions including a persistent cough and/or an asthma attack because of the unique mixture of bioflavonoid that the *passion fruit* contains and that has sedative and soothing effects.

Passion fruits is also recommended to people that have trouble sleeping because it reduces sleeplessness, restlessness and relieve anxiety.

N.137   *Dinner on the Level*   Yes / No

#lunch/dinner

pumpkin	1 cup
apple	2
cucumber	½ cup

HOW TO: chop cucumber and pumpkin in cubes and place it in your drinkable cup to measure. Juice the apples. Place everything in the blender and press START

TIPS: add ice cubes for freshness

ADD YOUR COMMENT: _____

_____

_____

N.138   *The Birthday Smoothie*   Yes / No

#dessert

crumbled pound cake	½ cup
strawberry	6
maple syrup	1 tbsp
strawberry syrup	1 tbsp
ground almond	1 tbsp
raspberry	1 handful
almond milk	½ cup
ice	4 cubes

HOW TO: place all the ingredients in the blender and press START

TIPS: it's your special day! pour the blend in a smoothie bowl and top with strawberry syrup and few raspberries

ADD YOUR COMMENT: _____

_____

_____

The intense passion

Yes / No

#breakfast/lunch

passion fruit	2
lime	½
banana	1
soy yoghurt	½ cup
soy milk	1 cup

HOW TO: place in a blender the milk, yoghurt and the banana peeled. Squeeze half of a lime inside the blender and add the pulp of two passion fruits. Press START to blend.

TIPS: you can use any dairy free alternative you rather opt for.

ADD YOUR COMMENT: _____

_____

_____

THE W@W FACTOR: *Soybean* or soya bean are a species of legume native to East Asia, now widely produced in United States and South America mainly for its edible bean which can be easily processed into a variety of food. They are usually green but they can be also yellow, brown or black.

In term of nutrients, *soybean* contains vitamin K, vitamin B6, vitamin C, riboflavin, folate, thiamin, iron, manganese, phosphorus, copper, potassium, magnesium, zinc, selenium and calcium. They are also a good source of organic compounds and antioxidants which gives *soybeans* a great variety of benefits. They help improve metabolism, increase healthy weight gain, defend against cancer, improve digestion, promote bone health, increase circulation, decrease the risk of diabetes and generally tone up the body. Furthermore, *soybean* are a source of healthier, unsaturated fat that helps lower the cholesterol level allowing, therefore, to prevent conditions like atherosclerosis which can lead to heart attack and stroke.

Soybean also help reduce the effects of the menopause in woman by been a great source of isoflavones, which are essential components of the female reproductive system. Isoflavones are able to bind to estrogen receptor cells so that the body doesn't notice the significantly drop of estrogen level during this time. It also helps to control symptoms of menopause such as mood swings, hot flashes and hunger pains.

N.140   <u>*The Super Man*</u>   *Yes / No*

#lunch

dates	1
figs	2
mandarin	2
avocado	½
apple	1 ½
almonds	1 handful
walnut	1 handful
wheat grass	1 tsp

HOW TO: juice mandarin and apple. Blend all the other ingredients together

TIPS: keep the mix refrigerated for 30 minutes.

ADD YOUR COMMENT: _____

_____
_____

N.141   _The Slim Plus_   Yes / No

#breakfast/lunch/dinner

green tea	¾ cup
ginger	15 ml
blueberries	1 handful
watermelon	~3 cubes
liquorice	1 stalk
maca powder	1 tbsp
ground coconut	1 tbsp
lemon	½

HOW TO: prepare the tea in advance. Juice the ginger and lemon. Blend all the ingredients together.

TIPS: store it in the fridge for around 30 minutes before to enjoy it.

ADD YOUR COMMENT: _____

_____

_____

Shades of the Sun   *Yes / No*
                     #**dinner**

orange	2
mango	1
carrot	2
ice cubes	3
spinach	1 handful

HOW TO: juice the oranges and the carrots. Chopped the mango in cubes and place it in the blender together with the spinach, the ice and all the juiced ingredients. Press START to blend.

TIPS: spirulina may be the right boost needed to be mix with this blend

ADD YOUR COMMENT: _____

_____

_____

THE W@W FACTOR: *Orange* is a fruit of the citrus family and is a hybrid between pomelo and mandarin. *Orange* trees are widely grown in tropical and subtropical climates for their sweet fruit and for the variety of possible use (eat fresh, dry or in aromatic candles and soaps).

About their nutritional value, one *orange* provide the 130% of vitamin C need for one day which make them a great boost for the immune system. It also contains vitamin A, vitamin B6, calcium, thiamin, riboflavin, niacin, folate, pantothenic acid, phosphorus, magnesium, manganese, selenium and copper. It also contains choline, zeaxanthin and carotenoids.

Research indicates that the citric acid and citrates from *oranges* may help prevent kidney stone formation. It also promote digestive health, lower the blood pressure, help fight cancer, support heart health and reduce risk of diabetes.

Furthermore, it fight skin damages caused by sun and pollution, reduce wrinkles and improve overall skin texture.

The Italian

#lunch

olives	3
tomato	1 large
oregano	a pinch
grated garlic	a pinch
salt	a pinch
zucchini	½
lettuce	5 leaves
grapes	6 yellow
orange	1
cucumber	¾

HOW TO: juice orange and cucumber. Blend all the ingredients together.

TIPS: add few ice cube in your smoothie glass

ADD YOUR COMMENT: _____

_____

THE W@W FACTOR: *Garlic* is a species in the onion genus, Allium. Native to Central Asia and northeastern Iran, it has a history of several thousand years of human consumption and use either as flavoring that as a traditional medicine.

Garlic is an excellent source of vitamin B6 and a good provider of manganese, selenium and vitamin C. In the garlic it is also possible to find traces of other minerals such as phosphorus, calcium, potassium, iron and copper. Eating garlic regularly it has been linked to reduce four of the major cause of death worldwide: stroke, heart diseases, cancer and infections. Garlic has been widely recognized as both a preventative agent and treatment of many cardiovascular and metabolic diseases, including atherosclerosis, hyperlipidemia, thrombosis, hypertension and diabetes. Most significantly, garlic help remove plaque buildup in arteries.

Furthermore, garlic is involved in reducing the high blood pressure by promoting the widening of blood vessels. Helps treating common cold, thanks to its antimicrobial, antifungal and antiviral properties.

Garlic is even involved in reducing hair loss: applying garlic, twice a day, on the scalp for three months as shown an improvement in hair grow!

Ultimately, garlic helps improve dementia symptoms: garlic contains antioxidant that can support body protective mechanisms against oxidative damage that can contribute to cognitive illness.

Marvel at the End

#lunch

yellow grapes	10
apricot	1
liquorice	1 stick
avocado	1
carrot	4 large
ginger	15ml
wheatgrass	1 tsp

HOW TO: juice carrots and ginger. Place all the other ingredients in the blender and press START

TIPS: you can easily swap wheatgrass with any other protein powder in you home.

ADD YOUR COMMENT: _____

_____

_____

THE W@W FACTOR: _Ginger_ is a flowering plant whose roots are widely used as spice or folk medicine. Ginger originated in the tropical rainforests from the Indian subcontinent to Southern Asia, arriving in Europe during the spice trade.

It contains vitamin C, vitamin B6, potassium, copper, manganese, magnesium, niacin, phosphorus and iron. It also contains gingerol, a compound with potent antioxidant and anti-inflammatory properties that has been linked to many unique health benefits as for its anti-cancer properties.

Ginger is perhaps better known to treat nausea and vomiting: also good for pregnant women fighting against their morning sickness! It has also powerful anti-fungal properties. It is involved in fighting stomach ulcers by decreasing levels of inflammatory proteins and blocking the activity of enzymes related to ulcer development.

Furthermore ginger, helps regulate blood sugar, relieve joint and muscle pain, lower cholesterol level, improves brain function and promote digestion.

The Purple Solution

#lunch

```
3
1
1 handful
1
~3-4 leaves
~6
~3
```

HOW .... eetroot and add all the ingredients to the blender. Press START to blen

TIPS: pl........ vocad. in the .... of the mix so that it will not stuck to the bottom. Check that the grapes .... seed. in it. .... all the seeds from the pear as well and chop it in small cubes.

ADD YOUR ....ME...

_____
_____
_____

THE W@W FAC.... .... plant native to the central Mediterranean region and widely cultivate......... etable.
About it nutritional va......... urce of vitamin K, vitamin C, vitamin A, folate, iron and copper. It als......... fiber, magnesium, zinc, phosphorus, vitamin B3, vitamin B1 and man.........
Parsley is used as a n......... diuretic, antiseptic and anti-inflammatory properties.
Furthermore, it is used to ....tes .... r, hypertension, cardiac disease, urinary disease, diabetes and variou......... a .... h bloating, gas, constipation, acid reflux and bad breath.
Parsley is a natural breath fresh......... is ills .... ria in the mouth that cause odours.

The One and All

#breakfast/lunch

acai berry	1 cube (frozen) or 1 tbsp (powder)
strawberry	6
banana	½
avocado	½
ice	5 cubes
green tea	¾ cup
spirulina	1 tsp
maca powder	1 tsp

HOW TO: prepare the green tea in advance. Defrost the acai berry until soft. Place all the ingredients in the blender and press START

TIPS: you can usually find the acai berry in powder or frozen. I like to use the frozen alternative because I believe it adds more flavour, but us up to you!

ADD YOUR COMMENT: _____

_____

_____

THE W@W FACTOR: Maca or Peruvian ginseng, is an edible herbaceous biennial plant, native to South America in the high Andes mountain of Peru. Commonly available in powder form or as a supplement. The main edible part of the plant is the root, which grows underground and that vary in colour, from white to black.

Maca root is a good source of carbs and proteins, is low in fat and contains a fair amount of fiber. It also contains vitamin C, vitamin B6, copper, iron, potassium and manganese.

Maca has been worldwide researched for its effects on the libido: it has been proved to increase sexual desire in either men and women. It also helps relieve symptoms of menopause including hot flashes and interrupted sleep. It has also been associated with reduce anxiety and symptoms of depression: mainly is involved in improving the mood!

Furthermore, the use of maca powder is very popular within athletes because helps gain muscle, increase strength, boost energy and increase exercise performance.

At last, when applied to the skin, maca may help protect it from the sun thanks to its polyphenol antioxidant and glucosinolates plant compound found in it.

A complex Machine *Yes / No*

#lunch/dinner

orange	2
cinnamon	1 tbsp
avocado	½
frozen berry	1 handful
flaxseed	1 tsp
ice	½ cup

HOW TO: juice the oranges. Place all the other ingredients in the blender and press START

TIPS: if you like turn this smoothie in your dinner by pouring it in a bowl and enjoy together with the family

ADD YOUR COMMENT: _____

_____

_____

THE W@W FACTOR: *Flaxseed*, also known as common flax or linseed, is a member of the genus Linum. It is a food and fiber crop cultivated in cooler region of the world. Grown since the beginning of civilization, flaxseeds are one of the oldest crops. There are two types, brown and golden, which are equally nutritious.

It contains protein, carbs, vitamin B1, vitamin B6, folate, calcium, iron, magnesium, phosphorus and potassium. Most of all, flaxseed contains Omega-3 essential fatty acid (the "good fats" related to many heart health benefits), lignans (with estrogen and antioxidant qualities that helps reduce the risk of cancer) and fiber (either soluble that insoluble, turning in more regular bowel movement). Flaxseed helps regulate blood sugar and lower cholesterol, lower blood pressure, aid in weight control.

Flaxseed are a great source of plant based protein: rich in the amino acids arginine, aspartic acid, and glutamic acid which help improve immune function, prevent tumours and has antifungal properties.

If you are vegan/vegetarian you should definitely add flaxseed to your diet!

Down with Love _Yes / No_

#lunch

avocado	1
peanut butter	1 tbsp
carrot	5
kale	1 handful
spirulina	1 tsp

HOW TO: juice only the carrots and then place it together with the rest of the ingredient in the blender.

TIPS: in the blender place the juice first, then the kale and then the peanut butter, spirulina and the avocado.

ADD YOUR COMMENT: _____

_____

_____

THE W@W FACTOR: _Spirulina_ is a spiral-shaped blue-green microalgae that grows in water lakes. Spirulina is the world's first superfood and one of the most nutrient-rich food on Earth. It is available on the market in both powder or tablet form.

It has between 55 and 70% of protein, vitamin B12, iron, calcium, phosphorus, beta-carotene, linoleic acid, arachidonic acid, gamma-linolenic acid, chlorophyll and phycocyanin, a pigment-protein that is found only in blue-green algae.

Spirulina is a natural detoxifier, oxygenetic the blood and helping cleanse the body of toxins and other impurities. It provides a near-instantaneous boost to one's energy, while helping to improve endurance and reduce fatigue. It helps improve the immune system, and provides exceptional support for the heart, liver, and kidneys.

Spirulina is also a natural appetite suppressant, and it helps to improve the body's digestive system. It also has very powerful antioxidant properties and it helps to balance the body's pH, reducing inflammation throughout the body.

Furthermore, spirulina helps prevent cancer, lower blood pressure, reduce cholesterol, lower the chances of a stroke, boost the memory, speed up weight loss and alleviates sinus issues, most specifically, it reduce itching, nasal discharge, nasal congestion and sneezing.

N.149   <u>Wash away</u>   *Yes / No*

#**dinner/snack**

lavender tea	¾ cup
watermelon cubes	½ cup
ground coconut	1 tbsp

HOW TO: prepare the lavender tea in advance. Place all the ingredients in the blender and press START

TIPS: add 3 ice cubes in the smoothie glass

ADD YOUR COMMENT: _____
_____
_____

THE W@W FACTOR: *lavender* or lavandula is a flowering plant in the mint family. Extensively produced in temperate climate areas as ornamental plant or culinary herbs or essential oil.
Lavender contains vitamin A (important to preserve healthy eye, reduce dryness of the eye, prevent cataract and night-blindness), calcium (for strong bone, keep osteoporosis at bay and release from premenstrual syndromes), iron (avoid symptoms of anemia, fatigue and other sickness due to a iron deficiency) and phytonutrients (for a overall health of your body).
It is used to treat anxiety and mental stress, helps ease migraine, treat acne when used as essential oil, ease joint and muscle pain, open the respiratory tract making easier to breath in people with cold and flu, helps control blood pressure.
Because of its stimulating nature, help with the urinary flow. and is a natural source of antioxidant.

A Cabbage a day Yes / No

#lunch

cabbage	3 leaves
potato	1 small
cucumber chunk	½ cup
soy milk	¾ cup
radish	2 leaves
black pepper	a pinch
salt	a pinch

HOW TO: boil the potato in advance. Prepare all the ingredients and blend it together.

TIPS: add 3 ice cubes in the smoothie glass

ADD YOUR COMMENT: _____
_____
_____

THE W@W FACTOR: *Cabbage* is a leafy green, red or white biennial plant grown for its dense-leaved heads. In the Middle Ages, Cabbage was a prominent part of the European cuisine. Even though cabbage is very low in calories, it has an impressive nutrients profile: vitamin K, vitamin C, vitamin B6, protein, fiber, folate, manganese, calcium, potassium, magnesium.

Cabbage also contains small amount of other micronutrients including vitamin A, iron and riboflavin. It contains powerful antioxidant as polyphenol and sulfur compounds.

Cabbage improve digestion, keep your heart healthy, fight inflammation, lower blood pressure, lower cholesterol level, avoid blood clotting, boost immunity, skin care, help with weight loss and prevent cataract by preventing macular degeneration thanks to the beta-carotene present in the cabbage.

Plus, improve brain health and hair care and speeds up healing thanks to the sulfur present in the cabbage which is a useful nutrient involved in fighting infections.

Go and smooth your cabbage NOW :-)

The horizon

#breakfast/lunch

turmeric	1 full tsp
hemp milk	¾ cup
banana	2 bananas
ice	4 ice cubes

HOW TO: place all the ingredients in the blender and press START to blend.

TIPS: place the turmeric powder on top of the ingredients or grate the turmeric and blend.

ADD YOUR COMMENT: _____

_____

_____

THE W@W FACTOR: *Hemp* milk, or hemp seed milk, is a plant based milk made from hemp seeds that are soaked and ground in water, yielding a milk flavored substance. It is one of the fastest growing plants and was one of the first plants to be spun into usable fiber 10,000 years ago. It can be refined into a variety of commercial items including paper, textiles, clothing, biodegradable plastics, paint, insulation, biofuel, food, and animal feed.

Hemp seeds are a great source of vitamin E and minerals such as phosphorus, potassium, sodium, magnesium, sulfur, calcium, iron and zinc. Hemp seeds contain over 30% fat. They are exceptionally rich in two essential fatty acids, linoleic acid (omega-6) and alpha-linolenic acid (omega-3). Hemp seeds are also a great source of arginine and gamma-linolenic acid, which have been linked with a reduced risk of heart disease. It may also relieve dry skin, improve itchiness, reduce symptoms associated with premenstrual syndrome (PMS), and may also positively affect symptoms of menopause.

Hemp seeds contain powerful antioxidants that the body needs to combat and fight against damaging molecules. Preventing cell damage can reduce the risk of cancer, heart disease, and other diseases.

Hemp seeds are rich in globulin, an important protein to synthesize antibodies which helps the body fight against infection.

For those with type 2 diabetes, or even at risk for diabetes, hemp seeds can help control blood glucose or sugar levels.

Ultimately, hemp seeds contain adequate amounts dietary fiber. Fiber plays a role in not only heart health, but can keep the digestive system working sufficiently and improve bowel regularity.

Digestive moments

#breakfast/lunch

banana	1
prune	2
cinnamon	1 tsp
almond butter	1 tbsp
almond milk	¾ cup

HOW TO: prepare all the ingredients and place it in the blender. Press START

TIPS: wash, chop and remove the stone from the prunes before to add it to the blend

ADD YOUR COMMENT: _____

_____

_____

THE W@W FACTOR: Prune is a dried plum, usually freestone cultivar (the pit is easy to remove). It is believed that the pruning process first began in Western Asia. By the 16th century the production of prune was very popular worldwide.

Prune contains vitamin A, C, E, K, potassium, calcium, copper, iron, magnesium, manganese, phosphorus, selenium, zinc, beta-carotene, proteins, fiber, folate and niacin.

Prunes are very beneficial in promoting a healthy vision as they provide up to 3% of the daily recommended value for vitamin A. They are also rich in carotene, which is an essential phytonutrient that helps boost overall eye health and prevent macular degeneration. Prunes are rich in antioxidants which prevent the onset of chronic illnesses such as cancer.

Furthermore, prune helps fight anemia, promove the cardiovascular health, boost immunity, relieves cramps, reduce the symptoms of constipation, reduce inflammation and infections in the body, promote bone health, promote healthy hair and healthy skin.

The shining Knight

#dinner

peach	1
pear	1
banana	1
honey dew melon	2 slices
carrot	3

HOW TO: place in the juicer the carrots and the melon. Add the juice to the blender together with the other ingredients carefully washed and chopped in small cubes.

TIPS: I would normally keep the skin on of peach and pear after been carefully washed and simply blend all together but is up to you to decide if take the skin off or leave it on.

ADD YOUR COMMENT: _____

_____

_____

THE W@W FACTOR: *peach* is an edible juicy fruit native to the region of Northwest China which is still one of the largest producer and where it represent a symbol of longevity and immortality.

About their nutrients, *peaches* are rich in vitamin A, beta-carotene,vitamin C, vitamin E, vitamin K, vitamin B1, B2, B3, B6, folate and pantothenic acid. Contains also minerals such as potassium, calcium, magnesium, iron, manganese, phosphorus, zinc and copper. They are low in calories, with no saturated fat or cholesterol and are a good source of dietary fiber.

Peaches helps to control obesity-related disease such as diabetes, metabolic syndrome and cardiovascular disease. It also promote skin care by reducing wrinkles, improve overall skin texture and help to fight skin damage caused by sun and pollution. Furthermore, *peaches* reduce risk of cancer, promote eye health, aids in digestion, maintains healthy nervous system, boost immunity, lower cholesterol level, improve cellular health. *Peaches* are valuable during pregnancy: the vitamin C helps in the healthy growth of the bones, teeth, skin, muscles, and blood vessels of the baby; the iron absorption is increased, which is crucial during pregnancy; the folate helps in preventing neural tube defects like spina bifida; the potassium helps in averting the muscle cramps and general fatigue and the presence of fiber aids in healthy digestion and reduces conditions like constipation.

The Chia solution

#breakfast

apricot	1
chia seed	1 flat tbsp
yoghurt	2 tbsp
banana	1
peach	1
spirulina	1 tsp
ice	½ cup

HOW TO: place all the ingredients in the blender and press START

TIPS: add water if necessary

ADD YOUR COMMENT: _____

_____

_____

THE W@W FACTOR: *chia* is the edible seed of Salvia hispanica, flowering plant in the mint family native to Central America. Chia seeds are oval, gray-coloured, with black and white spot. The seeds are hydrophilic, absorbing up to 12 times their weight in liquid when soaked and developing a mucilaginous coating that gives a distinctive gel texture.

Chia seeds are rich in Omega-3 fatty acid which makes it a MUST HAVE for who is embracing a plant based lifestyle. It also contains, protein, carbohydrates, fiber, manganese, phosphorus, calcium, zinc, copper and potassium. In smaller amount contains vitamin A, B, E and D, sulphur, iron, iodine, magnesium, niacin and thiamin. They are a rich source of antioxidant. Antioxidants speed up the skin's repair systems and prevent further damage.

The fiber presents in the chia are essential to regulate insulin levels, benefits bowel regularity and healthy stool. Helps with weight loss because, thanks to its fiber content, tent to make people feel full quickly because it absorb a considerable amount of water and immediately expands in the stomach when eaten. Omega-3 works to protect the heart by lowering blood pressure, bad cholesterol and inflammation. Also, helps with diabetes treatment, boost energy level and restore the metabolic functions, provide stronger bones, build muscle, fight breast and cervical cancer and helps with dental health by maintaining your teeth strong and keeping the bad breath germs away!

N.155   *Lemonland*   *Yes / No*

#dessert

lemon zest	of 1 lemon
lemon juice	of 1 lemon
dairy free vanilla ice cream	2 tbsp
cinnamon	1 flat tbsp
banana	1
water	½ cup

HOW TO: prepare all the ingredients and blend it together

TIPS: plain still water will do, but if you enjoy extra texture go for sparking

ADD YOUR COMMENT: _____

_____

_____

N.156   *Dirty Green*   *Yes / No*

#dinner

mint	3 leaves
cucumber	1
ice	4 cubes
strawberry	5

HOW TO: juice only the cucumber and then pour the juice with the rest of the ingredients in the blender. Press START

TIPS: is a perfect drink for a afternoon snack. Light and fresh, fill with goodness

ADD YOUR COMMENT: _____

_____

_____

Did I Hear Acai?   *Yes / No*

#breakfast/dessert

acai berry(frozen)	1 square
apple	3
banana	1
coconut yoghurt	1 tbsp
ice	3 cubes

HOW TO: juice only the apple and add all the other ingredient to the blender mixed with the juice.

TIPS: take the acai berry out of the freezer a good half an hour earlier to gain a smooth consistency. Option to leave it in hot water for a couple of minutes.

ADD YOUR COMMENT: _____

_____

_____

THE W@W FACTOR: *Acai berry* is a small, round, deep purple fruit obtained from the acai palm tree. It is one of the most nutritious berries on the planet. Also called the Amazonian palm berry, *acai* is native to the Amazon rainforest.

Acai berries is loaded on nutrient: it contains Vitamin C, Vitamins A, B1, B2, B3 and E, calcium, magnesium, zinc and copper. It also contain amino acids which help promote muscle performance, energy production, endurance and strength. It is naturally high in essential fatty acids which promote heart health and a healthy nervous system.

The fibre found in *Acai berry* skin and pulp can aid digestion. Fibre can help prevent or relieve constipation and may help support a healthy cardiovascular system.

Furthermore, in the *Acai* there is a very high concentration of antioxidants which is involved in preventing free radical damage.

More benefits of this berry are: promote skin health, aids weight loss, reduce irritation, improve cellular health, has anti-aging effect, boost energy, improve mental function and optimize the cholesterol level.

<u>A Sweet Red</u> *Yes / No*

#**dinner**

raspberry	1 cup
cranberry	½ cup of juice
pomegranate	1 handful
cucumber cubes	½
agave syrup	1 tsp
ice	5 cubes

HOW TO: prepare your ingredients and place it in the blender. Press START

TIPS: in buying your cranberry juice choose the one with less sugar content

ADD YOUR COMMENT: _____

_____

_____

THE W@W FACTOR: *Cranberries* are a group of evergreen dwarf shrubs that can be found in Central and Northern Europe as throughout the northern United States, Canada and Chile, it depends of the variety.

The flowers are dark pink, with very distinct reflexed petals, leaving the style and stamens fully exposed and pointing forward. The fruit is a berry that is larger then the leaves of the plant and is initially green, turning red when ripe. It is edible but with and acidic taste that overwhelms its sweetness. Most cranberries are processed into products such as juice, sauce, jam and sweetened dried cranberries.

Cranberries are low in calories and rich in vitamin C, vitamin A, vitamin K, vitamin E, manganese, fiber and copper. They are a good source of antioxidant which protect our cells from free radical damage.

Cranberries prevent and treat urinary tract infections, decreases inflammation, may help prevent cancers, improves immune function, benefits the digestive tract and reduce risk of heart disease.

The good soil gift

#lunch

green olives	4
black beans	1 tbsp
oregano	a pinch
salt	a pinch
carrot	4
banana	1

HOW TO: prepare all the ingredients and blend it

TIPS: use pre cooked beans to speed the preparation

ADD YOUR COMMENT: _____

_____

_____

THE W@W FACTOR: *olive* is a species of small tree in the family Oleaceae, cultivated in many places and considered naturalized in all the countries of the Mediterranean coast. The olive's fruit, also called the olive, is of major agricultural importance in the Mediterranean region as the source of the olive oil: one of the core ingredients in the Mediterranean cuisine.

Olives are a good source of several vitamins and minerals such as vitamin E, iron, copper, calcium, sodium, carbs and fiber, fatty acid (oleic acid) and many other plant compound that makes the olive extremely rich in antioxidant.

Dietary antioxidant have been shown to reduce the risk of chronic diseases such as heart disease and cancer. It may reduce oxidative damage and help fight infections caused by bacteria.

Furthermore, it helps regulate cholesterol level, improve bone health, prevent blood clots, protect against anaemia, boost immune system, keep skin soft and healthy reducing the appearance of wrinkles by 20% thanks to the oleic acid action.

The maple art!
#breakfast

banana	1 and a half
soy vanilla yoghurt	4 tbsp
maple syrup	1 tsp
turmeric powder	1 tsp
ice	½ cup

HOW TO: place all the ingredients in the mixer and press START to blend

TIPS: if you like have a more liquid consistency add soy milk or apple juice to your mix.

ADD YOUR COMMENT: _____

_____

_____

THE W@W FACTOR: *Maple syrup* is a syrup made from the maple tree. It was first collected and used by the indigenous peoples of North America, and the practice was adopted by European settlers, who gradually refined production methods. Technological improvements in the 1970s further refined syrup processing. The Canadian province of Quebec is by far the largest producer, responsible for 70 percent of the world's output.

The nutrients found in *maple syrup* include energy, water, protein, fat, carbohydrates, and sugars. In terms of minerals, it contains calcium, iron, magnesium, phosphorus, sodium, potassium, and zinc. Vitamins such as thiamin, riboflavin, niacin, and B6 are also found in this syrup.

There are many beneficials outcome by using *maple syrup* such as an improved heart health, a stronger immune system, a easier digestion, a stabilized blood sugar level, and a help in fight inflammatory diseases.

The consumption of *maple syrup* also helps in maintaining male reproductive health. There are certain minerals such as zinc, in *maple syrup*, that are useful for a healthy reproductive system, particularly the prostate gland. Reduction in the level of the minerals increases the risk of disorders, such as prostate cancer.

Deeply simple

#lunch

strawberry	7
avocado	1
agave syrup	1 tsp
soy milk	¾ cup

HOW TO: prepare all the ingredients and blend it together

TIPS: add 4 ice cubes in the smoothie glass

ADD YOUR COMMENT: _____

_____

_____

THE W@W FACTOR: *Agave syrup*, or Agave nectar, is a sweetener commercially produced from several species of Agave. Agave is a flowering plant from the hot and arid regions of Mexico and Southwester United States. The plants are perennial but each group of leaves, flowers once and then dies.

Being a relative new product on the market, relatively few researches have been done so far.

But be careful not to overuse this syrup because even though in its original natural form agave plant contains strong antioxidant and anti-inflammatory properties, none of this beneficial properties are present in the agave sold in the market. This is because agave syrup it is actually manufactured using a highly processed procedure that basically strips the naturally occuring agave juice of all nutritional value. Shockingly, the finishing product contains a very high amount of fructose that makes it potentially dangerous for the health if used regularly and in high portions.

Therefore, until new extracting process are created use your agave syrup in minimum amount, the high level of fructose means that you need very little quantity to sweeten your smoothie, or opt for an alternative syrup. Right now, the healthier on the market appear to be date sugar.

Date sugar, *because it is made from dried, pulverized dates, rather than undergoing a refinement process, is actually a whole food and thus retains all the vitamins and minerals found in dates.*

The Unexpected

#lunch/dinner

orange	2
lime zest	of 1 lime
ginger zest	~15 gr
papaya	1
dragon fruit	½
chestnut	3
fig	1

HOW TO: juice the orange. Add then all the ingredients in the blender and mix together with the juice base.

TIPS: add a couple of ice cubes or keep it refrigerated for a fresher mix

ADD YOUR COMMENT: _____

_____

_____

THE W@W FACTOR: *Chestnut* or Castanea belong to the family Fagaceae, which also includes oaks and beeches. The four main species are commonly known as European, Chinese, Japanese, and American chestnuts. The fruit is contained in a spiny (very sharp) cupule 5–11 cm in diameter, also called "bur" or "burr". The burrs are often paired or clustered on the branch and contain one to seven nuts. Around the time the fruits reach maturity, the burrs turn yellow-brown and split open in two or four sections.

Chestnuts have one of the highest content of dietary fiber in the world of "nuts". In it, we can also find vitamin C, copper, magnesium, potassium, good fat, nutrients, antioxidant and vitamin B -complex (folate, riboflavin, thiamine).

It may seem like an average, everyday nut, but chestnut have a number of important health benefits including their ability to improve digestive health, strengthen bones, manage diabetes, protect cardiovascular health, boost the immune system, and lower blood pressure. They also increase cognition and prevent chronic illnesses.

Word of Caution: many people suffer from tree nut allergies of varying severity, so be cautious when adding a new nut such as chestnut to your smoothie.

A Green Date...
#breakfast/lunch

dates	3
spinach	1 handful
kale	1 handful
almond milk	¾ cup

HOW TO: place all the ingredients in the mixer and press START to blend

TIPS: add a protein shake to the mix to boost the energetic value such as wheat-grass

ADD YOUR COMMENT: _____

_____

_____

THE W@W FACTOR: *Kale* or leaf cabbage ia a certain type of cabbage grown for their edible leaves. It can have green or purple coloured leaves.

Raw kale is composed of 84% water, 9% carbohydrates, 4% protein, and 1% fat. It contains a large amount of vitamin K, and in smaller amount vitamin A, vitamin C, vitamin B6, folate, manganese, thiamin, riboflavin, pantothenic acid, vitamin E and several dietary minerals, including iron, calcium, potassium, and phosphorus.

Boiling raw kale diminishes most of these nutrients, while values for vitamins A, C, and K, and manganese remain similar.

Kale has many benefits which includes: anti-inflammatory properties, antioxidant properties, improve eye health, detoxifies the body, boost heart health, fortifies the bones, lower risk of cancer and protect infant brain development.

As fresh as a Basil

#lunch/dinner

basil	2 leaves
tomato	1 large
pear	1
beetroot	2
ice	½ cup
lemon	½

HOW TO: juice lemon and beetroot. Blend all the ingredients together.

TIPS: wash and dice the tomato in 4 parts. Remove then the top central part because it doesn't blend properly.

ADD YOUR COMMENT: _____

_____

_____

THE W@W FACTOR: *Basil* is a culinary herb of the family Lamiaceae (mints). It is native to tropical regions from central Africa to Southeast Asia. It is a tender plant, and is used in cuisines worldwide.

Basil is sensitive to cold, with best growth in hot, dry conditions.

It is known to be an anti-inflammatory, anti-bacterial and powerful adaptogen — meaning it helps the body to respond to stress and fight disease. It also contains vitamin C, vitamin A, vitamin K and manganese.

Basil helps balance acid within the body and restore the body's proper pH level. This can improve digestion and immunity by helping healthy bacteria flourish within the gut microflora, while also decreasing harmful bacteria that can cause disease. Basil has also been used to help reduce bloating and water retention, loss of appetite, stomach cramps, acid reflux, and even to kill stomach worms or parasites.

Basil is also considered an antidepressant by some since it can positively impact brain function within the adrenal cortex, helping stimulate neurotransmitters that regulate the hormones responsible for making us happy and energetic. promoting healthy blood pressure.

Furthermore, basil supports liver function, helps detoxify the body, protects from diabetes and fights against the metabolic syndrome.

The aroma of basil is believed to increase libido and arousal, possibly by increasing blood flow and energy level, while reducing inflammation.

Fantastic 5...   Yes / No
                    #lunch/dinner

mandarin	2
pomegranate	1 handful
avocado	½
lime	½
cucumber	½

HOW TO: juice cucumber and mandarin. Place all the ingredients in the blender and press START

TIPS: if you don't have available a fresh pomegranate, go for the juice filling ⅓ of your cup.

ADD YOUR COMMENT: _____
_____
_____

THE W@W FACTOR: _Mandarin_ is a small citrus tree with fruit resembling other oranges, usually eaten plain or in fruit salads. Mandarins are sweet, juicy and easy to peel. The leaves are shiny and green, rather small. The fruit color is orange, orange-yellow, or orange-red. Their shape is spherical or oblate. The fruits may be seedless or contain a small number of seeds.
China is the bigger producer of mandarin worldwide.
The fruits contain a large amount of sugar (up to 10.5%), vitamins C, B1, B2, provitamin A, free organic acids, phytoncides, lectins, and mineral salts, potassium, manganese and magnesium. It also contains dietary fiber.
Mandarin have been proved to lower the risk of liver cancer, improve cholesterol, help with weight loss, protect vision and support the immune system.
Also, mandarin help build bone strength, create new bone, and fight osteoporosis. It helps lower blood pressure and keep blood flow moving smoothly.
Ultimately, mandarin are great for the health of your skin.

@It's complicated@ Yes / No

#lunch/dinner

kale	1 handful
papaya	1
cantaloupe melon	1 thick slice
spinach	1 handful
ice	5 ice cubes
parsley	~5 leaves

HOW TO: juice the melon and add it to the mixer together with the other ingredients

TIPS: maybe add a little <u>sparkling water</u> for a twist in the taste

ADD YOUR COMMENT: _____
_____
_____

THE W@W FACTOR: *Cantaloupe* melon refer to the orange-fleshed kind of melon. Originally produced in India and Africa, took the name from Europe, sees now China as one of the largest producer worldwide.

Cantaloupe is rich in nutrients: includes vitamin A, beta-carotene, vitamin B1, B2, B6, B9, vitamin C, vitamin K plus many minerals like potassium, calcium, iron, magnesium, phosphorus and zinc.

It has many health benefits like improves vision, boosts immunity, reduces dehydration, prevents asthma, prevents cancer, regulates blood pressure, controls diabetes, promotes digestion, treats arthritis and help in hair and skin care.

Starry Night
#**lunch/dinner**

rocket	5 leaves
lettuce	2 leaves
avocado	½
parsley	3 leaves
sparkling water	¾ cup
pear	1 small

HOW TO: prepare all the ingredients, wash it, chop it and blend it together

TIPS: reduce the amount of rocket if you find the flavour too strong

ADD YOUR COMMENT: _____

_____

_____

THE W@W FACTOR: *Rocket* or arugula is an edible annual plant in the Brassicaceae family used as a leaf vegetable for its fresh peppery flavor. Native to the Mediterranean region, it belong to the same family of broccoli, kale, and brussels sprouts. Arugula grows to a height of 20-100 centimeters and is recognizable by its small and white flowers.

All in all, arugula is a low-calorie, nutrient-rich food. It contains: vitamin A, vitamin K and vitamin C, folate, calcium, protein and fat. It is packed with carotenoids, as well as many other minerals like potassium, manganese, iron, and calcium, all of which are beneficial and necessary elements in a person's diet. Also, arugula contains phytochemicals, which are beneficial in preventing cancer.

Arugula has a wealth of health benefits. It's involved in decreases the risk of obesity, diabetes, heart disease, and overall mortality while promoting a healthy complexion, increased energy, keep the mind clear and focused and help in weight loss.

Lifestyle plus

#breakfast

strawberries	5
granola	1 tbsp
banana	½
agave syrup	1 tbsp
spinach	1 handful
avocado	⅓
apple	2

HOW TO: juice the apples and blend everything together

TIPS: the quality of the fruit and veg is very important. Shop local and try to buy from reliable sources

ADD YOUR COMMENT: _____

_____

_____

THE W@W FACTOR: _Granola_ is a breakfast food and snack food consisting of rolled oats, nuts, honey or other sweeteners such as brown sugar, and sometimes puffed rice. Dried fruit, such as raisins and dates, and confections such as chocolate are sometimes added.

Granola is often eaten in combination with yoghurt, honey, fresh fruit, milk or other forms of cereal.

It also serves as a topping for various pastries, desserts or ice cream.

Granula was invented in Dansville, New York, by Dr. James Caleb Jackson at the Jackson Sanitarium in 1863: a prominent health spa that operated into the early 20th century on the hillside overlooking Dansville.

The food and name were revived in the 1960s, and fruits and nuts were added to it to make it a health food that was popular with the health and nature-oriented hippie movement.

The long list of health benefits commonly attributed to granola is mainly due to its dictary fibre. The minerals in it include sodium, potassium, zinc, phosphorus, magnesium, calcium, and iron. Vitamins include vitamin E, vitamin C, niacin, vitamin E, and thiamin.

Granola, particularly if it includes flax seeds, is often used to improve digestion.

It gives relief from constipation and excess flatulence; prevent overeating and helps in managing weight; aids in digestion and diabetes management; reduce risk of cancer and anaemia; reduce blood pressure; reduces harmful cholesterol; protects skin against harmful effects of sunburn; boost energy level and cognitive function in the body.

<u>**A Full Boost**</u> *Yes / No*

#**breakfast**

coffee powder	1 tbsp
soy milk	1 cup
ice	5 cubes
cookies	3

HOW TO: place all the ingredients in the mixer and press START to blend

TIPS: use your favourite cookie to mix with it. I would rather have plain breakfast cookies but your choice.

ADD YOUR COMMENT: _____

_____

_____

THE W@W FACTOR: *Coffee* is a brewed drink prepared from roasted coffee beans, which are the seeds of berries from the Coffee plant. People first started to grow coffee in subtropical areas in Africa as well as some islands in Southern Asia. This beverage is seen as a rich source of caffeine. However, it is its high content of antioxidants that contributes to the health benefits of the coffee: mainly polyphenols.

Additionally, coffee also incorporates a number of micronutrients such as magnesium, niacin, manganese, riboflavin, potassium and sodium, etc. One of the most well-known benefits of coffee is positive effects on brain function.

Acting as a stimulant, caffeine can block adenosine function – an inhibitory neurotransmitter – and promote the activity in brain.

Also, this substance may help with tiredness, improves mood, enhance vigilance as well as cognitive function.

Furthermore, studies have found coffee having a positive impact in fighting type 2 diabetes, liver cancer, heart diseases, depression, promote weight loss and increase physical performance.

Breeze that Freeze

#dessert

dairy free vanilla ice cream	3 tbsp
green tea	1 cup
honey dew melon	1 cup of cubes
ice	4 cubes

HOW TO: prepare the tea in advance and blend everything together.

TIPS: ideal for a beauty friends sleepover

ADD YOUR COMMENT: _____

_____

_____

THE W@W FACTOR: *Green tea* is a type of tea that is made from *Camellia sinensis* leaves. Green tea originated in China, but its production and manufacture has spread to many other countries in Asia.

Several varieties of green tea exist, which differ substantially based on the variety of *C. sinensis* used, growing conditions, horticultural methods, production processing, and time of harvest.

Green tea is the healthiest beverage on the planet.

It is loaded with antioxidants and nutrients that have powerful effects on the body.

It has catechins, the astringency component of the green tea which, with its antibacterial and antioxidant effect, is involved in decreasing blood pressure, reducing body fat, preventing cancer, preventing tooth decay, lowering cholesterol level, reducing glycemic level and fighting bad breath bacteria.

It has caffeine, the bitterness component of the tea, which helps decrease tiredness and drowsiness, increase stamina, hangover prevention, and work as a mild diuretic.

It has Theanine, the full-bodied flavour component in the tea, involved in neuronal cell protection, relaxation effect and lowering blood pressure.

Vitamin C, B2, folic acid, beta-carotene, vitamin E, all present in the green tea, work for the maintenance of healthy skin and mucous membrane, helping with night time vision and as prevention of arteriosclerosis.

Mineral as potassium, calcium, phosphorus and manganese, which are biological regulators, are all present in this kind of leaves.

It also contains saponins (anti influenza effect), fluorine (prevention of tooth decay), y-aminobutyric acid (lower blood pressure), chlorophyll (deodorizing effect). Green tea is a wonder of nature!

Matcha day

#lunch

dairy free vanilla ice cream	3 tbsp
matcha	1 tsp
spinach	1 handful
blueberry	1 handful
ice	½ cup
water	½ cup

HOW TO: place all the ingredients in the blender and press START

TIPS: wash carefully all the fruit and veg to eliminate traces of pesticide. We allow only goodness in our body!

ADD YOUR COMMENT: _____

_____

_____

THE W@W FACTOR: *Matcha* it's a finely ground powder of specially grown and processed green tea leaves. The preparation of matcha starts several weeks before harvest and may last up to 20 days, when the tea bushes are covered to prevent direct sunlight. This slows down growth, stimulates an increase in chlorophyll levels, turns the leaves a darker shade of green, and causes the production of amino acids, in particular theanine.

Matcha tea is rich in fiber, chlorophyll and vitamins C and A. It also provides selenium, chromium, zinc, magnesium and potassium.

Matcha tea contains a unique, potent class of antioxidant known as catechins, which aren't found in other foods. In particular, the catechin EGCg (epigallocatechin gallate) provides potent cancer-fighting properties.

Most importantly, EGCg and other catechins counteract the effects of free radicals from the likes of pollution, UV rays, radiation, and chemicals, which can lead to cell and DNA damage. Since over 60% of the catechins in matcha are actually EGCg, a daily matcha regimen can help restore and preserve the body's integral well-being and balance.

Matcha is also rich in L-Theanine, a rare amino acid that actually promotes a state of relaxation and well-being by acting upon the brain functioning. And while L-Theanine is common in all tea, matcha may contain up to five times more of this amino acid than common black and green teas. As an additional benefit, L-Theanine may help memory and learning abilities, while inhibiting any possible side-effects from caffeine, a natural component of green tea.

Therefore, a bowl of matcha promotes concentration and clarity of mind without any of the nervous energy found in coffee.

Take me by Surprise///   Yes / No

#**lunch/dinner**

cucumber	1
peach	1
ginger	20ml
pear	1
ice	2 cubes

HOW TO: juice only the cucumber and then place all the ingredients in the mixer and press START to blend

TIPS: play with the amount of fruit to adjust the sweetness of the blend

ADD YOUR COMMENT: _____

_____

_____

THE W@W FACTOR: As crazy as it sound *cucumber*, even though is perceived, prepared and eaten as a vegetable, is actually a fruit. Originally from South Asia, now grows on the global market.

Cucumber is rich in vitamin K, also known as clotting vitamin for its essential role in fighting against blood clot formations.

It also contains vitamin A, vitamin C, folate, phosphorus, magnesium, calcium and potassium. Most importantly cucumbers are 95.2% water which helps maintaining your body hydrated.

Also, cucumber supports heart health, protects the brain from neurological diseases, protects the skin from aging, fights inflammation in the body, reduces the risk of cancer, relieves pain, reduces bad breath, prevents constipation and helps maintaining a healthy body weight.

Vitamin Plus   *Yes / No*

#breakfast/lunch/dinner

beetroot	2
orange	1
banana	1
pineapple	1 slice

HOW TO: juice beetroot and orange. Blend everything together.

TIPS: cut a slice of pineapple in small cubes and place it in your measure cup. Half cup is all you need.

ADD YOUR COMMENT: _____

_____

_____

THE W@W FACTOR: *Beetroot* is the tap root portion of the beet plant, usually known in North America as the beet, also table beet, garden beet, red beet, or golden beet. From the Middle Ages, beetroot was used as a treatment for a variety of conditions, especially illnesses relating to digestion and the blood. Belonging to the same family as chard and spinach, both the leaves and root can be eaten - the leaves have a bitter taste whereas the round root is sweet. Typically a rich purple colour, beetroot can also be white or golden.

Beetroot is of exceptional nutritional value: it is rich in calcium, iron and vitamins A and C. Beetroot are an excellent source of folic acid and a very good source of fibre, manganese, iron, copper, magnesium and potassium. Beetroot fibre has been shown to increase the number of white blood cells, which are responsible for detecting and eliminating abnormal cells.

Health benefits of beetroot includes lower blood pressure, protect the heart, prevent cancer, protect the liver, boost energy level, fights inflammation, promotes brain health, control blood sugar, aids digestion, reduces bad cholesterol, helps treat anaemia, promotes strong bones and teeth, aids weight loss, it has anti-aging properties, improve skin health and prevent osteoporosis

Furthermore, beetroot are a great source of carotenoids that can reduce the risk of cataract formation and prevent age-related macular degeneration.

Red beetroot have been ranked as one of the 10 most potent antioxidant vegetables and are also one of the richest sources of glutamine, an amino acid, essential to the health and maintenance of the intestinal tract.

Get ready for the Night   Yes / No
#lunch

celery	3 stalks
apple	1
kale	1 handful
avocado	1
parsley	~7 leaves

HOW TO: juice celery and apple. Mix the juice together with the kale, avocado and parsley and enjoy

TIPS: if you believe the blend is to thick for your taste, simply reduce the amount of avocado in the mix

ADD YOUR COMMENT: _____

_____

_____

THE W@W FACTOR: _Apple_ is a sweet, edible fruit, belonging to the apple tree, Malus Domestica, and originated in Central Asia.
It is now cultivated worldwide.

Apples are extremely rich in antioxidant that help to protect our cell from free radical damage caused by pollution, smoke, inflammation within the body, etc.

It also contains dietary fibre needed to support a healthy digestive system, vitamin A and vitamin C to improve the immune system, vitamin K fighting blood clotting, vitamin B7 that helps break down fat and iodine which is involved in healthy thyroid function.

They are also very filling despite their low calories content which makes it ideal for weight control. Remember: an apple a day keeps the doctor away!

N.175   *Dracula*   Yes / No

#lunch

grated garlic	1 small
spinach	2 handful
beetroot	2
carrot	3
salt	a pinch

HOW TO: wash properly all the ingredients. Then place it in a blender a press START

TIPS: a little amount of garlic is enough to gain a lovely intense flavour. Begin with blend just a small portion...you may always add some more later on.

ADD YOUR COMMENT: _____

_____

_____

N.176   *Peperonata*   Yes / No

#lunch

red bell pepper	1
beetroot	1
kale	1 handful
apple	1
orange	1

HOW TO: place all the ingredients in the blender and press START

TIPS: clean properly the red pepper, open it in half and remove all the seeds before to blend.

ADD YOUR COMMENT: _____

_____

_____

Open Your Eyes   Yes / No

#breakfast

cinnamon	1 tbsp
soy vanilla milk	¾ cup
banana	1
coffee powder	1 tbsp
raspberry	1 handful
ice	2 cubes

HOW TO: place all the ingredient in the mixer and press start

TIPS: is a perfect mix to energise your morning. Don't miss out!

ADD YOUR COMMENT: _____

_____

_____

THE W@W FACTOR: *Cinnamon* is a spice obtained from the inner bark of several tree. The potent smell and unique flavor come from a compound called cinnamaldehyde, which has powerful medicinal properties.

From the nutritional value point of view, it contains vitamin K, calcium, iron, manganese and dietary fibre. Cinnamon contains more active antioxidants than garlic, oregano, and other seasoning.

It possess anti-inflammatory properties that helps your body repair tissue damage and fight infections.

Reduce the risk of heart disease, combat bacterial infection, fight diabetes, protect from developing neurological disorders, lower chance of cancer, promote dental health and fresher breath.

Apple salt

#lunch/dinner

lettuce	3 leaves
cucumber	½
banana	1
apple	1 ½
pinch of salt	
ice	4 cubes

HOW TO: juice the apple and the cucumber. Blend all the ingredients together.

TIPS: make sure all your vegetables and fruits are properly washed

ADD YOUR COMMENT: _____

_____

_____

THE W@W FACTOR: *Lettuce* is an annual plant of the daisy family, Asteraceae. It is most often grown as a leaf vegetable but also for its stem and seeds. Europe and North America originally dominated the market for lettuce, but by the late 20th century the consumption of lettuce had spread throughout the world.

Despite its reputation for being a complete zero on the nutritional scale, iceberg lettuce provides significant amounts of vitamins A (a powerful antioxidant that helps to maintain night vision and eye health and supports cell growth) and vitamin K (a vitamin that works with calcium to prevent bone fractures and that is integral for blood clotting).

It also provides calcium (which keeps bones and teeth strong, supporting at the same time muscle function, nerve function and blood clotting), potassium (a mineral that reduces blood pressure by lessening the effects of salt in the diet), vitamin C (a powerful antioxidant that helps keep your immune system healthy), and folate (a B-vitamin that helps to make DNA and genetic material. It's especially important for women who are pregnant or who are planning to become pregnant).

Although it's low in fiber, it has a high water content, making it a refreshing choice during hot weather.

Apple Lego   Yes / No

                              #breakfast

apple	2 ½
dairy free soy yoghurt	2 tbsp
blueberry	½ cup
oats	1 tbsp
banana	½

HOW TO: juice the apples. Add all the ingredients in the blender and press START

TIPS: choose golden apples for a sweeter and more fulfilling taste

ADD YOUR COMMENT: _____

_____

_____

THE W@W FACTOR: *Oats* sometimes called the **common oat**, is a species of cereal grain grown for its seed, which is known by the same name. Oats are best grown in temperate regions. They have a lower summer heat requirement and greater tolerance of rain than other cereals. In 2016, global production of oats was 23 million tonnes, led by Russia with 21% of the world total.

Oats are loaded with important vitamins, minerals and antioxidant plant compounds. Oat contains manganese, phosphorus, magnesium, copper, iron, zinc, folate, vitamin B1 (thiamin) and vitamin B5 (pantothenic acid). It also held smaller amounts of calcium, potassium, vitamin B6 (pyridoxine) and vitamin B3 (niacin). This is coming with carbs, protein, fat and fiber, with little calories.

This means that oats are among the most nutrient-dense foods you can eat.

Also, whole oats are high in antioxidants and beneficial plant compounds called polyphenols: mainly avenanthramides, which are almost solely found in oats. Avenanthramides may help lower blood pressure levels by increasing the production of nitric oxide which helps dilate blood vessels and leads to better blood flow. In addition, avenanthramides have anti-inflammatory and anti-itching effects.

Furthermore, oats are high in the soluble fiber beta-glucan, which has numerous benefits: it helps reduce cholesterol and blood sugar levels, promotes healthy gut bacteria, increases feelings of fullness and relieve constipation by regulating bowel movements.

Din Don Dan   *Yes / No*
                          #lunch/dinner

yellow bell pepper	2
white cucumber	½
cucumber	½
apple	1
banana	1
ice	½ cup

HOW TO: juice only the apple. Cut in chunks the cucumber and the white cucumber. Slice up the yellow pepper. Place the banana with all the other ingredients in the mixer and press START

TIPS: add an energy powder of your choice

ADD YOUR COMMENT: _____

_____

_____

THE W@W FACTOR: *Bell Pepper* also known as sweet pepper or capsicum are native to Mexico, Central America and northern South America. Imported to Spain in 1493, will soon be spread to the entire Europe and Asia. They come in every colour: green, yellow, orange and red.
Bell peppers are an excellent source of vitamin A, vitamin C, potassium, folic acid and fibre. It helps boost metabolism as well as reduces the appetite, which in the long run helps with the weight loss.
Packed with antioxidant and anti-inflammatory benefits, it reduces 'bad' cholesterol, controls diabetes, brings relief from pain and eases inflammation.
Bell peppers also contain vitamin B6, which is essential for the health of the nervous system and helps renew cells.
The bell pepper is a good source of Vitamin E, which is known to play a key role in keeping skin and hair looking youthful, strong and healthy.

#beachside

Yes / No

#lunch/dinner

almond butter	2 tbsp
tomato	3 large
carrot	3
flaxseed	1 tsp

HOW TO: juice carrots and tomato. Blend all together.

TIPS: keep it refrigerated for 30 minutes and stir thoroughly before to drink.

ADD YOUR COMMENT: _____

_____

_____

THE W@W FACTOR: *Almond* is a species of tree native to Mediterranean climate regions of the Middle East. Almond is also the name of the edible and widely cultivated seed of this tree.

The almond is a very popular tree nut. Despite being high in fat, they are highly nutritious and extremely healthy. Almonds are high in healthy mono-unsaturated fats, fibre, protein and various important nutrients: vitamin E, manganese, magnesium, copper, vitamin B2 (riboflavin) and phosphorus.

Almonds are a fantastic source of antioxidants that helps to protect against oxidative stress, which can damage molecules in cells and contribute to ageing and diseases like cancer. Those powerful antioxidants in almonds are largely concentrated in the brown layer of the skin.

Other health benefits of the almonds includes: blood sugar control, blood pressure level, cholesterol level control, hunger control and calories intake control.

Flax a seed

#**breakfast**

cashew nuts	1 handful
almond milk	¾ cup
soy yoghurt	2 tbsp
figs	1
papaya	½
flaxseed	1 tsp

HOW TO: soak the cashew nuts in advance. Place all the ingredients in the blender and press START

TIPS: cashew nuts can even simply be left in water overnight or cook in boiling water for 15 minutes and then run under cold water before to blend.

ADD YOUR COMMENT: _____

_____

_____

THE W@W FACTOR: *Papaya* is a small, sparsely branched tree, usually with a single stem growing from 5 to 10m tall, with spirally arranged leaves confined to the top of the trunk.

The fruit is a large berry about 15–45 cm long and 10–30 cm in diameter. It is ripe when it feels soft (as soft as a ripe avocado or a bit softer) and its skin has attained an amber to orange hue. Native to Mexico and northern South America, papaya has become naturalized throughout the Caribbean Islands, Florida, Texas, California, Hawaii, and other tropical and subtropical regions of the world.

Papaya is rich in antioxidant nutrients such as carotene, flavonoids, and vitamin C, as well as vitamin B (folate and pantothenic acid). It is also a good source of fiber and minerals such as magnesium. Together, these nutrients help improve cardiovascular health and protect against colon cancer.

The health benefits of papaya also includes: ease digestion, promote weight loss, regulate menstruation, prevent infections, provide relief from a toothache, help in skin care, improve heart health, reduce the symptoms of acne and burns, prevent macular degeneration, help in treats constipation, help prevent arthritis and boost the immune system.

N.183   *The Big Chunk*   *Yes / No*

#dinner

water	¾ cup
pear	1
banana	1
carrot	1 large size chopped in tiny parts

HOW TO: prepare tiny chunk of carrot, banana and pear. Place then the ingredients into the mixer and add the water

TIPS: if the carrot is to hard for your blender, cook it first for 5 to 10 minutes: just enough to soften the carrot. Pass it under cold water and then add it to the mix.

ADD YOUR COMMENT: _____

_____

_____

N.184   *Gelato with the Twist*   *Yes / No*

#dessert

apple	2 ½
dairy free Ice cream	2 tbsp
kale	1 handful
banana	1

HOW TO: juice the apples and then place the juice in the blender together with the other ingredients and press START

TIPS: if you like feel more energised add a tsp of spirulina powder to your glass and stir.

ADD YOUR COMMENT: _____

_____

_____

Jalapeno Love   Yes / No

#lunch

jalapeno pepper	½
ice	4 cubes
beetroot	½
dairy free soy yoghurt	1 tbsp
hemp milk	¾ cup
spinach	1 handful
parsley	3 leaves
mint	3 leaves
maple	1 tsp

HOW TO: Blend all the ingredients together

TIPS: carefully wash all the veggie before to blend

ADD YOUR COMMENT: _____

_____

_____

Out of Bed

#breakfast

turmeric	1 tsp
coconut water	¾ cup
oats	1 tbsp
mix nuts	1 tbsp
banana	½
ice	3 cubes
peanut butter	1 tbsp
dates	1
vanilla	1 tsp

HOW TO: add all the ingredients in the list in your blender and press START

TIPS: It is a rich breakfast alternative. Great especially if you have an intense day ahead and you know you are going to need lots of energy.

ADD YOUR COMMENT: _____

_____

_____

The Rose Taste

#snack/dinner

green tea	¾ cup
raspberry	½ cup
mint	3 leaves
banana	½

HOW TO: prepare the green tea in advance. Wash and place all the other ingredients in the blender together with the tea and press START

TIPS: for a quick ice tea preparation, pour a little hot water in a cup together with a tea bag. Use a tea spoon to push the extract out for a minute. Take the tea bag out and add cold water and ice cubes

ADD YOUR COMMENT: _____

_____

_____

THE W@W FACTOR: *Raspberry* is the edible fruit of a multitude of plant species in the genus *Rubus* of the rose family. Rich in colour and with a sweet juicy taste. Wild raspberries are believed to have originated in Asia, but there are also varieties of raspberries that originated in the USA. Currently, the leading producers of raspberries include Poland, Germany, Yugoslavia, Russia, Chile, and the United States.

Raspberries are excellent sources of vitamin C, manganese, and dietary fiber. They are also rich in B vitamins, folic acid, copper, and iron. They have the highest concentration of antioxidant strength amongst all fruits. This is due to its high concentration of ellagic acid, anthocyanins, gallic acid, quercetin, cyanidin, catechins, pelargonidin, kaempferol and salicylic acid.

Because of this, *raspberries* can be considered as one of the best natural treatments for cancers.

The health benefits of raspberries include their ability to aid in weight loss, improve skin health, and strengthen the immune system. The oil from raspberries has a sun protection factor. Raspberries work like magic on wrinkles. Relieves nausea in pregnant woman. Helps in production of milk in lactating mother. Protects against fungal and bacterial infections. And is beneficial in regulating menstrual cycle in women.

I feel gorgeous

#**lunch/breakfast**

mango	½
ice	3 cubes
coconut yoghurt	1 tbsp
banana	1
pineapple	½
blueberry	1 handful
cinnamon	1 tsp

HOW TO: juice only the pineapple and then mix all the ingredients together

TIPS: is the perfect smoothie to share with your friends during your mani-pedi. Poor it in a fancy glass ;-)

ADD YOUR COMMENT: _____

_____

_____

THE W@W FACTOR: *Pineapple* is a tropical plant with an edible fruit cultivated mainly in Costa Rica, Brazil and Philippine. Pineapples are naturally high in fibre, an important component of a healthy diet that can help improve digestion.

Pineapples also contain a good array of vitamins and minerals including calcium, manganese, vitamins A and C, as well as folic acid.

One of the key phytonutrients found in *pineapple* is bromelain that has long been recognised for its anti-inflammatory and anti-microbial effects. It helps to reduce the risk of cardiovascular conditions such as thrombosis by helping to prevent blood clotting. Improve wound healing. Boost the immune system, and respiratory health, aiding digestion and strengthening bones.

It also helps in reducing inflammation, curing coughs and colds, and accelerating weight loss.

Black World

#lunch/dinner

blackberry	½ cup
dairy free vanilla ice cream	3 tbsp
beetroot	½
fig	1
apple	2 ½

HOW TO: juice only the apples. Blend all the ingredients!

TIPS: if you don't have a juicer, use plain water instead of the apples.

ADD YOUR COMMENT: _____

_____

_____

THE W@W FACTOR: *Fig* is an Asian species of flowering plant in the mulberry family, known as the **common fig** (or just the **fig**). Native to the Middle East and western Asia, it has been sought out and cultivated since ancient times and is now widely grown throughout the world, both for its fruit and as an ornamental plant.

The health benefits of *figs* come from the presence of minerals, vitamins, and fiber contained in the fruits. They contain a wealth of beneficial nutrients, including vitamin A, vitamin B1, vitamin B2, calcium, iron, phosphorus, manganese, sodium, potassium, and chlorine. That high concentration of fiber helps to promote healthy, regular bowel function and prevents constipation. The fiber in figs helps also reduce weight and is often recommended for obese people. However, their high-calorie count can also result in weight gain: a few are enough to get the recommended amount of nutrients, so don't overeat. Furthermore, *figs* help to keep the cholesterol level under control.

The natural chemicals in *fig* leaves make them an ideal component for a tea base. Fig leaf tea has been popularly prescribed for various respiratory conditions like bronchitis and is also used as a way to prevent and lessen the symptoms of asthma. *Figs* are rich in calcium, which is one of the most important components in strengthening bones and reducing the risk of osteoporosis. They are also rich in phosphorus, which encourages the bone formation and spurs regrowth if there is any damage to or degradation in bones. The high mucilage content in figs helps heal and protect sore throats. The soothing nature of these fruits and their natural juices can relieve pain and stress on the vocal cords as well.

It's a new day

#snack

lime	1
turmeric powder	1 tsp
mix protein powder	1 tsp
apple	2

HOW TO: juice only the apple. Squeeze one lime straight into the blender add the apple juice and then add the powders.

TIPS: keep it in the fridge before to drink it or add some ice to add a refreshing taste

ADD YOUR COMMENT: _____

_____

_____

THE W@W FACTOR: *lime* is a hybrid citrus fruit, which is typically round, lime green, 3–6 centimetres in diameter, and contains acidic juice vesicles. Predominantly known for its ascorbic acid reserves, *lime* provides 32% of the daily recommended vitamin C intake.

It has high water content and a good source of minerals like calcium, iron, copper, sodium, magnesium, phosphorus, and potassium as well as vitamins like folate, vitamin A, vitamin E, and vitamin K.

Moreover, *lime* peel and pulp are also rich in dietary fiber, antioxidants, flavonol glycosides like kaempferol, as well as diverse phytochemicals like polyphenols, limonene, and terpenes.

The health benefits of *lime* include weight loss, improved digestion, reduced respiratory disorders, enhanced immunity, relief from constipation, as well as prevention from cancer and kidney stones.

It also aids in skin care, hair care, and eye care.

N.191   *Macau Meravigliau*   *Yes / No*

#dinner/snack

maca mix with water	¾ cup
coconut yoghurt	2 tbsp
banana	1
blueberry	½ cup

HOW TO: fill a glass with cold spring water and pour a tsp of maca powder in it. Stir well! Place all the ingredients in the blender and press START

TIPS: add a couple of ice cubes in your smoothie cup for an invigorating sensation

ADD YOUR COMMENT: _____

_____

_____

N.192   *Blue as Gold*   *Yes / No*

#dinner

blueberries	½ cup
mango	1 ½
mint	2 leaves
agave syrup	1 tsp
parsley	2 leaves

HOW TO: juice the mango and then place it in the blender with the rest of the ingredients and press START

TIPS: have it fresh! Add a couple of ice cubes straight in your glass

ADD YOUR COMMENT: _____

_____

_____

Soul Searching

#lunch/dinner

spirulina	1 tsp
dairy free vanilla ice cream	2 tbsp
kiwi	3
spinach	1 handful
pear	1
ice	½ cup

HOW TO: juice the kiwis and then blend everything together.

TIPS: this smoothie is quite thick. If you like it more juicy add some water.

ADD YOUR COMMENT: _____

_____

_____

THE W@W FACTOR: *Kiwifruit* (often abbreviated as *kiwi*), or Chinese is the edible berry of several species of woody vines in the genus *Actinidia*. It has a fibrous, dull greenish-brown skin and bright green or golden flesh with rows of tiny, black, edible seeds. The fruit has a soft texture, with a sweet and unique flavor. China produced 56% of the world total of kiwifruit.

Kiwi is an excellent source of vitamin C (ascorbic acid). Other vitamins including vitamin A, folate, vitamin E (alpha-tocopherol), and vitamin K (phylloquinone) are also present in good amounts. The mineral wealth of kiwi includes a tremendous quantity of potassium along with other minerals such as calcium, magnesium, and phosphorous. All these vital nutrients in the fruit come with an added bonus of dietary fiber.

Health benefits of kiwi include skin care, improved cardiovascular health, lower blood pressure, and prevention of strokes. It also aids in the treatment of cancer, insomnia, macular degeneration, and diabetes. Due to the flavonoid-rich compounds found in kiwi, it also helps during pregnancy and promotes the absorption of iron in the body. Besides, the anti-microbial properties of kiwi guard against a range of pathogens and strengthen the immune system. Due to the great antioxidant and vitamin C content in kiwi fruit, it is known to treat asthma. It improves lung function and also prevents wheezing among children.

Love me Like you do

#lunch

broccoli	50 gr
coconut yoghurt	2 tbsp
avocado	1
coconut milk	½ cup

HOW TO: place all the ingredients in the blender and press start

TIPS: increase or reduce the amount of broccoli in order to gain a stronger or softer flavour

ADD YOUR COMMENT: _____

_____

_____

THE W@W FACTOR: *broccoli* is an edible green plant in the cabbage family whose large flowering head is eaten as a vegetable. *Broccoli* was first introduced to the United States by Southern Italian immigrants, but did not become widely popular until the 1920s. *Broccoli* is a great source of vitamins K and C, a good source of folate (folic acid) and also provides potassium, fiber.

Vitamin K is essential for the functioning of many proteins involved in blood clotting Vitamin C is involved in the build of collagen, which forms body tissue and bone, and helps cuts and wounds heal. It is also a powerful antioxidant and works to protect the body from damaging free radicals.

Fiber promote digestive health and help lower cholesterol.

Potassium is a mineral and electrolyte that is essential for the function of nerves and heart contraction.

Folate is necessary for the production and maintenance of new cells in the body.

The Love Maker

Yes / No

#breakfast/dinner

strawberry	8
pineapple	~ ½ (¾ cup of juice)
cacao powder	1 tbsp
cinnamon	1 tsp

HOW TO: juice only the pineapple. Blend then all the ingredients.

TIPS: place the smoothie in a fancy glass and top with soy whipped cream, cacao and cinnamon stick and share it with your loved one

ADD YOUR COMMENT: _____

_____

_____

THE W@W FACTOR: *cocoa bean* or just *cocoa*, which is also called the *cacao bean* or *cacao*, is the dried and fully fermented seed of *Theobroma cacao*, from which cocoa solids and, because of the seed's fat, cocoa butter can be extracted. The beans are the basis of chocolate, The cacao tree is native to the Amazon Basin. The three main varieties of cocoa plant are Forastero, Criollo, and Trinitario. The first is the most widely used, comprising 80-90% of the world production of cocoa. Cocoa beans of the Criollo variety are rarer and considered a delicacy. One of the largest producers of Criollo beans is Venezuela (Chuao and Porcelana). Trinitario (from Trinidad) is a hybrid between Criollo and Forastero varieties. It is considered to be of much higher quality than Forastero, has higher yields, and is more resistant to disease than Criollo. Immature cocoa pods have a variety of colours, but most often are green, red, or purple, and as they mature, their colour tends towards yellow or orange.

Cocoa is rich in minerals such as iron, magnesium, calcium, phosphorus, copper, and manganese. It is also a good source of selenium, potassium, and zinc while providing the body with carbohydrates, protein, and dietary fibers. In addition to this, the cholesterol content in it is almost negligible. It contains cocoa butter, which is a mixture of monounsaturated fats like oleic acid and saturated fats, namely stearic acid and palmitic acid. Health benefits of cocoa include relief from high blood pressure, cholesterol, obesity, constipation, diabetes, bronchial asthma, cancer, chronic fatigue syndrome, and various neurodegenerative diseases. It is beneficial for quick wound healing, skin care, and it helps to improve cardiovascular and brain health. It also helps in treating copper deficiency. It possesses mood-enhancing properties and exerts protective effects against neurotoxicity.

Cacao beans contain xanthine and theophylline, which aid in relaxing bronchial spasms and opening constricted bronchial tubes. This facilitates an easy flow of air and is valuable in curing various allergies, including asthma and shortness of breath.

The Cheeky Pea

#lunch

chickpeas	1 tbsp
avocado	½
broccoli	3 small pieces
apple	2 ½
lime	½

HOW TO: juice the apples and the lime. Place all the other ingredients in the blender together with the juice base and press START

TIPS: keep the blend refrigerated for around 30 minutes and give it a good stir before to drink it.

ADD YOUR COMMENT: _____

_____

_____

THE W@W FACTOR: *Chickpea* is a legume of the family Fabaceae, It is one of the earliest cultivated legumes and 7500-year-old remains have been found in the Middle East. *Chickpeas* are a type of pulse, with one seed pod containing two or three peas. It has white flowers with blue, violet, or pink veins. There are roughly 90 identified species of chickpea, although the most common variants are pale-brown, black, green, and red chickpeas.

Chickpeas or garbanzo beans are a powerhouse of nutrients, packed with plant-based protein, dietary fiber, and carbohydrates. They are a rich source of antioxidants and minerals such as iron, zinc, magnesium, folate, and phosphorous. The nutty seeds also have a number of essential vitamins like thiamin, riboflavin, niacin, vitamin C, A, B6, B12, and vitamin K.

Chickpeas are an excellent source of plant-based protein which helps prevent diabetes and aid in weight loss. The amazing benefits of chickpeas include the ability to improve digestion, prevent heart diseases, stabilize blood pressure levels, and lower the risk of genetic diseases and cancer. They also boost bone, skin, and hair health.

Consuming garbanzo beans can be a safe and natural way to counter menopausal and postmenopausal symptoms like night sweats, mood swings, and hot flashes. *Chickpeas* contain plant hormones known as phytoestrogens, which mimic the body's natural female hormone estrogen. They also guard against diseases that commonly affect women such as breast cancer and osteoporosis.

Gentle on the Skin   Yes / No

#breakfast

blueberry	1 handful
oat yoghurt	2 tbsp
acai berry	1 frozen
mango	1 juiced

HOW TO: juice the mango and then add all the ingredients to the blender

TIPS: make it a regular smoothie for a most efficient result on the skin

ADD YOUR COMMENT: _____

_____

_____

THE W@W FACTOR: *blueberries* are perennial flowering plants with blue or purple coloured berries. Native to North America, they were introduced in Europe in the 1930s. Blueberries are an excellent source of antioxidants that are very powerful in preventing disease and improving all bodily.

The anthocyanin, vitamin A, vitamin C, vitamin E, selenium, copper, magnesium, and phosphorus in these powerful fruits can help prevent cognitive damage and heal neurotic disorders. This combination of nutrients prevents the death of neurons and protects the health of the central nervous system.

Blueberries health benefits include improving cognitive function, treating urinary tract infection, preventing cancer, slowing aging process, fighting diabetes, supporting healthy heart, promoting healthy immunity, enhancing the skin, supporting healthy eyes, and reducing risk of high blood pressure

Plum me up!

#dinner

pomegranate	2 tbsp
agave syrup	1 tsp
plum	3 juiced
ice	¾ cup
lemon	½
fennel	½

HOW TO: juice the fennel, the lemon and the plums.

TIPS: add more fennel if you need extra juice base for your smoothie. Pomegranate can either be blend or juice.

I know is a lot of hard work to peel the pomegranate but the taste is totally worth it.

ADD YOUR COMMENT: _____

_____

_____

THE W@W FACTOR: *Fennel* is a flowering plant species in the carrot family. It is a hardy, perennial herb with yellow flowers and feathery leaves. It is indigenous to the shores of the Mediterranean but has become widely naturalized in many parts of the world, especially on dry soils near the sea-coast and on riverbanks.

Fennel, which has the scientific name *Foeniculum vulgare miller*, or its essence, is widely used around the world in mouth fresheners, toothpaste, desserts, antacids, and in various culinary applications.

Vitamin C, A, folate, potassium, manganese and calcium, dietary fibre, carbohydrate and proteins can all be found in the fennel.

The health benefits of *fennel* include relief from anaemia, indigestion, flatulence, constipation, colic, diarrhoea, respiratory disorders, and menstrual disorders. It also aids in eye care.

Furthermore, it inhibits growth of cancerous tumours, increase brain function and cognitive abilities, maintains cholesterol level, reduces high blood pressure and prevent premature ageing.

<u>Washing the sins away</u>   *Yes / No*

#lunch

sparkling water	¾ cup
spinach	1 handful
kale	1 handful
avocado	1
mint	~5 leaves

HOW TO: add all the ingredients to the blender

TIPS: opt for still water for a less bubbling taste

ADD YOUR COMMENT: _____

_____

_____

THE W@W FACTOR: why *water* is so important for a human body? Each molecule in *water* contains one oxygen and two hydrogen atoms. There are no calories and fat content found in it. The adult body is made of about 60% water.

Your body needs an adequate amount of *water* to function properly as your brain, blood, and bones are composed of high water content.

The health benefits of drinking *water* includes preventing osteoporosis, balancing body temperature, assist with breathing, support metabolism, relieves pain and support cardiovascular health. Other benefits includes dissolving kidney stones, preventing arthritis, supporting pregnancy, improving skin condition, balancing PH levels, promoting digestion and supporting removal of excretory. Drinking *water* helps maintain the balance of body fluids.

The functions of these bodily fluids include digestion, absorption, circulation, creation of saliva, transportation of nutrients, and maintenance of body temperature. *Water* helps energize muscles. Cells that don't maintain their balance of fluids and electrolytes shrivel, which can result in muscle fatigue.

Coffee Break   *Yes / No*
                        #breakfast

cold coffee	1 or 2 shots
maple syrup	1 tsp
ice	½ cup
kale	1 handful
avocado	½
pear	1

HOW TO: prepare the coffee and decide if today you need only one shot of espresso or 2 if is going to be a difficult day. Mix your shot with cold water enough to refill one cup. Place all the ingredients in the blender and press START

TIPS: this smoothie drink/bowl is a great substitute of your lunch break. Take it with you at work!

ADD YOUR COMMENT: _____
_____
_____

Veggie Mania   Yes / No

#lunch

yellow paprika	1
chickpeas	1 tbsp
cucumber	1
avocado	½
black pepper	a pinch
salt	a pinch

HOW TO: juice the cucumber. Chop and blend all the ingredients

TIPS: pour it in a bowl and enjoy a perfect dinner

ADD YOUR COMMENT: _____

_____

_____

The Crazy Olive

Yes / No

#lunch

dates	2
grapes	5 yellow
soaked cashew nuts	1 handful
almond milk	¾ cup
olives green	5

HOW TO: leave the cashew nuts soaking overnight in cold water. Mix all the ingredients together and press START

TIPS: eat it as a lunch alternative. It works great!

ADD YOUR COMMENT: _____

_____

_____

THE W@W FACTOR: The *cashew tree* is a tropical evergreen tree that produces the cashew seed and the cashew apple. It can grow as high as 14 m (46 ft), but the dwarf cashew, growing up to 6 m (20 ft), has proved more profitable, with earlier maturity and higher yields.

The species is originally native to north eastern Brazil. The *cashew* nut, often simply called a cashew, is widely consumed. It is eaten on its own, used in recipes, or processed into cashew cheese or cashew butter. The cashew apple is a light reddish to yellow fruit, whose pulp can be processed into a sweet, astringent fruit drink or distilled into liquor.

Cashews are very nutritious and are a powerhouse of proteins and essential minerals including copper, calcium, magnesium, iron, phosphorus, potassium, and zinc. Sodium is also present in very small quantities. *Cashews* also contain vitamins such as vitamin C, vitamin B1 (thiamin), vitamin B2 (riboflavin), vitamin B3 (niacin), vitamin B6, folate, vitamin E (alpha-tocopherol), and vitamin K (phylloquinone). They are a source of oleic acid and provide a good quantity of monounsaturated fat and low amounts of polyunsaturated fats with no harmful cholesterol if consumed appropriately. The health benefits of cashews include a healthy heart, strong nerve and muscle function, aid in the formation of red blood cells, and an improved bone and oral health. They also provide relief from diabetes, anaemia, and gallstones. By offering an antioxidant defence, they also encourage a better immune system.

Oil extracted from *cashew* seeds is widely used for curing cracked heels. Powdered cashew seeds have anti-venom effects and are used for treating snake bites.

<u>A Savour Day</u>   *Yes / No*

#dinner

parsley	~8 leaves
celery	2 sticks
grapefruit	1
ice	3
lemon	1

HOW TO: juice grapefruit, celery and lemon and mix with ice and the parsley

TIPS: don't have a juicer? Place all the ingredients in the mixer and add little water

ADD YOUR COMMENT: _____

_____

_____

THE W@W FACTOR: *lemon* is a species of small evergreen tree in the flowering plant family Rutaceae, native to Asia.

The health benefits of *lemon* include treatment of indigestion, constipation, dental problems, throat infections, fever, internal bleeding, rheumatism, burns, obesity, respiratory disorders, cholera, and high blood pressure, while also benefiting your hair and skin. Known for its therapeutic property since generations, *lemon* helps strengthen your immune system, cleanse your stomach, and is considered a blood purifier.

Lemon juice, especially, has several health benefits associated with it. It is well known as a useful treatment for kidney stones, reducing strokes, and lowering body temperature. As a refreshing drink, lemonade helps you stay calm and cool.

The health benefits of *lemon* are due to its many nourishing elements like vitamin C, vitamin B6, vitamin A, vitamin E, folate, niacin, thiamin, riboflavin, pantothenic acid, copper, calcium, iron, magnesium, potassium, zinc, phosphorus, and protein. It is a fruit that contains flavonoids, which are composites that contain antioxidant and cancer-fighting properties.

The Biggest Lunch   Yes / No

#lunch

lentil	1 tbsp
potato	1 small
sparkling water	½ cup
pear	1 small
cucumber	½
salt	a pinch
ginger	~15 ml

HOW TO: boil the potato in advance with a pinch of salt. Juice the cucumber and ginger. Place everything together in the blender and press START

TIPS: buy the ready to eat lentils to make it easier for you otherwise remember to cook the lentil in the advance and rinse it then under cold water.

ADD YOUR COMMENT: _____

_____

_____

THE W@W FACTOR: *Lentil* are an edible legume and the oldest pulse crop known, and among the earliest crops domesticated in the Old World, having been found as carbonized remains alongside human habitations dating to 11,000 BCE in Greece. The origins of *lentils* are in the Near East and Central Asia. The popular kinds of lentils include black lentils, red lentils, brown lentils, mung bean, yellow split peas, yellow lentils, macachiados lentils, French green lentils, black-eyed pea, kidney beans, soya beans, and many more varieties. Each country has its own native group of lentils, which are more or less similar and provide the same benefits. One very good way to have *lentils* is after they have sprouted because they contain methionine and cysteine. These two amino acids are very significant in muscle-building and strengthening of our body. Methionine is an essential amino acid that is supplied through the food, and cysteine is a non-essential amino acid that can then be synthesized. *Lentils* contain the highest amount of protein originating from any plant. The amount of protein found in lentils is up to 35%, which is comparable to red meat, poultry, fish, and dairy products. Lentils contain carbohydrates (15-25 grams per 100 grams). They are a good source of dietary fiber and also have a low amount of calories. Other nutritious components found are molybdenum, folate, tryptophan, manganese, iron, phosphorus, copper, vitamin B1, and potassium. The health benefits of *lentils* include improved digestion, a healthy heart, diabetes control, cancer management, weight loss, prevention of anemia, and better electrolytic activity due to potassium and is great for pregnant women. It also aids in the prevention of atherosclerosis and in maintaining a healthy nervous system.

The Greatest Love

#breakfast/dessert

cherry	6 pitted
dairy free vanilla ice cream	2 tbsp
liquorice	1 stick
fig	2
Hemp milk	¾ cup

HOW TO: mix all the ingredients together and press START

TIPS: if you have available try to use amarena cherry for a even sweeter taste.

ADD YOUR COMMENT: _____

_____

_____

THE W@W FACTOR: *Cherry* is the fruit of many plants of the genus *Prunus*, and is a fleshy drupe (stone fruit). The *cherry* fruits of commerce usually are obtained from cultivars of a limited number of species such as the sweet cherry (*Prunus avium*) and the sour cherry (*Prunus cerasus*). The name 'cherry' also refers to the cherry tree. They are eaten all around the world.

Cherry has unique antioxidant profile, combined with vitamin E, vitamin A, vitamin C, zinc, quercetin, phenolic compounds, and even certain useful hormones. It is also rich in carbs, fiber, proteins, fat, manganese, potassium, and copper. The antioxidants it is most well-known for are anthocyanins, which are anti-inflammatory and immune-boosting in nature.

Calcium, iron, magnesium, omega 3, and omega 6 fatty acids are also present in this fruit in smaller quantities.
They have a huge amount of benefits. **Cherry** protects against diabetes; promotes better sleep; decreases belly fat; helps ward off alzheimer's; reduces risk of stroke; slows the aging of skin; reduces muscle pain; helps regulate blood pressure; helps with osteoarthritis relief and helps to prevent colon cancer.

<u>The Family Lunch</u>   *Yes / No*

#lunch/dinner

carrot	2
apple	1
banana	2
ice	3
spinach	1 handful

HOW TO: juice apple and carrot and then blend it with the rest of the ingredients

TIPS: may be too rich in banana flavour so in case banana is not your favourite fruit reduce the amount of it or change it with one avocado.

ADD YOUR COMMENT: _____
_____
_____

THE W@W FACTOR: *Banana* is an edible fruit, probably first domesticated in Papua New Guinea is now produced in most of the Countries around the world with India and China as largest producer. The fruit is variable in size, colour and firmness but is usually elongate and curved, with soft flesh rich in starch covered with a rind that may be yellow, green, red, purple or brown when ripe. This fruit grows in clusters hanging from the top of the plant. *Bananas* contains a variety of vitamins and minerals which includes vitamin B6, manganese, vitamin C, potassium, dietary fiber, protein, magnesium, folate, riboflavin, niacin, vitamin A, iron. *Bananas* also contain tryptophan, an amino acid that studies suggest plays a role in preserving memory and boosting your mood.

The high level of potassium in the *banana* helps maintain fluid level in the body and regulates the movement of nutrients and waste products in and out of cells.

Potassium also helps muscles to contract and nerve cells to respond. It keeps the heart beating regularly and can reduce the effect of sodium on blood pressure.

Potassium may reduce the risk of kidney stones forming as people age. In turn, healthy kidneys make sure that the right amount of potassium is kept in the body.

In general, *bananas* may help prevent asthma, cancer, high blood pressure, diabetes, cardiovascular disease, and digestive problems.

N.207 *No Stop* Yes / No

#lunch

cherry	6 pitted
grapes	3 pitted
kiwi	1
avocado	½
apple	1
cucumber	½
amarena cherry syrup	1 tsp

HOW TO: juice the kiwi, apple and cucumber. Blend everything together

TIPS: add few ice cubes straight in your smoothie glass

ADD YOUR COMMENT: _____
_____
_____

N.208 *Avocado Mania* Yes / No

#lunch

avocado	1 ½
salt	a pinch
lemon	½
carrot	2
apple	½

HOW TO: juice the carrots, lemon and apple. Place the juice in the blender together with salt and avocado and press START

TIPS: when choose the avocado to buy opt for soft one with dark skin.

ADD YOUR COMMENT: _____
_____
_____

<u>**On with the odd**</u>

#breakfast

tahini sauce	1 tbsp
peanut butter	1 tbsp
almond milk	¾ cup
banana	1

HOW TO: place all the ingredient in the blender and press START

TIPS: no need to drink it….pour it in a bowl and scoop right in

ADD YOUR COMMENT: _____

_____

_____

THE W@W FACTOR: *tahini* sauce is a condiment made from toasted ground hulled sesame. *Sesame* is a flowering plant widely naturalized in tropical regions around the world and is cultivated for its edible seeds. These seeds are considered the oldest oilseed crop in the world and have been cultivated for more than 3,500 years. Evidence of their native forms in Africa and India. The health benefits of *sesame* seeds are due to their nutritional content, including vitamins, minerals, natural oils, and organic compounds which consist of calcium, iron, magnesium, phosphorus, manganese, copper, zinc, fiber, thiamin, vitamin B6, folate, protein, and tryptophan. *Sesame* seeds are extremely beneficial for health but are often overlooked. They have the ability to prevent diabetes, lower blood pressure, prevent a wide variety of cancers, build strong bones, protect against radiation, and improve the heart health. They also help cure sleep disorders, improve digestion, reduce inflammation, boost respiratory health, and aid in dental care. These powerful seeds improve blood circulation, detoxify the body, and eliminate depression and chronic stress.

N.210   _The Milky Way_   Yes / No

#breakfast

maple syrup	1 tsp
soy yoghurt	2 tbsp
muesli	1 tbsp
almond milk	¾ cup
banana	½
tahini	1 tbsp

HOW TO: blend everything together.

TIPS: is a morning smoothie. Prepare it for breakfast or lunch…
avoid dinner time, is a heavy alternative for so late in the day

ADD YOUR COMMENT: _____
_____
_____

N.211   _The Old Goodness_   Yes / No

#dinner

apple	1 ½
orange	1 ½
banana	1
ice	5

HOW TO: juice apple and orange and then blend with banana and ice.

TIPS: add a protein powder of your choice for extra energy

ADD YOUR COMMENT: _____
_____
_____

As fresh as the Nature

#dinner

watermelon	1 slice
spinach	1 handful
pear	1
banana	1

HOW TO: juice the watermelon and mix it with the other ingredients

TIPS: for extra thickness add ½ extra banana

ADD YOUR COMMENT: _____

_____

_____

THE W@W FACTOR: *watermelon* is a scrambling and trailing vine of the flowering plant. There is evidence from seeds in Pharaoh tombs of watermelon cultivation in Ancient Egypt. *Watermelon* is grown in tropical and subtropical areas worldwide for its large edible fruit, also known as a *watermelon*, which is a special kind of berry with a hard rind and no internal division.

Significant amounts of vitamin C, calcium, magnesium, fiber, protein, and a large amount of potassium are found in the *watermelon*. Furthermore, they contain vitamin A, vitamin B6, niacin, thiamin, and a wide variety of carotenoids and phytonutrients, including lycopene!

The health benefits of *watermelon* include prevention of kidney disorders, high blood pressure, cancer, diabetes, heart diseases, heat stroke, macular degeneration, and impotence. Arginine, present in watermelon, is beneficial in curing erectile dysfunction, and the stimulating nature of the chemical can boost the libido, reduce frigidity, and give your love life a fresh start after you enjoy a few slices of watermelon together!

N.213   _The Shining Blend_   Yes / No

#dinner

passion fruit	1
banana	½
ice	4
carrot	3 large

HOW TO: juice the carrots. Place the juice in the blender together with all the other ingredients and press START

TIPS: add agave syrup if you find the mix not sweet enough for your palate. Add a pinch of salt if you like to have a more savoury flavour.

ADD YOUR COMMENT: _____

_____

_____

N.214   _A Jump in the Sea_   Yes / No

#snack/dinner

watermelon	1 slice
avocado	½
kiwi	1

HOW TO: juice the watermelon. Get enough juice to fill up your smoothie cup of ¾. Blend then all the ingredients together.

TIPS: add 4 ice cubes in your smoothie cup

ADD YOUR COMMENT: _____

_____

_____

N.215   _A New Beet_   Yes / No

#lunch

beetroot	3
blueberry	½ cup
coconut yoghurt	2 tbsp
banana	½
mix nuts	1 handful

HOW TO: juice the beetroot. Blend everything together.

TIPS: if you find the beetroot flavour to strong, add only one beetroot and add plain water.

ADD YOUR COMMENT: _____
_____
_____

N.216   _A Smooth Skin_   Yes / No

#dessert

coconut ice cream	2 tbsp
pineapple	¾ cup of juice
banana	½
vanilla syrup	4 drops
ice	3 cubes

HOW TO: juice the pineapple until getting one cup full of juice. Add all the ingredients in the blender and press START

TIPS: if you don't have a juicer, go for water base with a couple of pineapple cubes to add to your blend

ADD YOUR COMMENT: _____
_____
_____

N.217 *Tea Mania* *Yes / No*

#snack/dinner

green tea   ½ cup
cantaloupe melon   1 cup of cubes
avocado   1

HOW TO: prepare the tea in advance. Blend all the ingredients together

TIPS: is a very thick blend. It is better to pour it in a smoothie bowl and enjoy with a spoon. If you rather drink it, reduce the avocado of half and use only half cup of melon in cubes

ADD YOUR COMMENT: _____
_____
_____

N.218   *Matcha Plus*   *Yes / No*

#breakfast

matcha   1 tsp
coconut yoghurt   3 tbsp
blueberry   1 handful
banana   ½

HOW TO: stir 1 tsp of matcha powder into ¾ cup of cold plain water. Place all the ingredients in the blender and press START

TIPS: add few ice cubes in the glass

ADD YOUR COMMENT: _____
_____
_____

N.219   _Guilt Free Butter_   Yes / No

#all times good

dates	1
soy yoghurt	2 tbsp
almond butter	1 tbsp
cucumber	1
ice	3 cubes

HOW TO: juice the cucumber and then blend all the ingredients together

TIPS: turn it in a smoothie bowl. It is actually perfect for every meal: have it for breakfast, lunch or dinner. You can never go wrong!

ADD YOUR COMMENT: _____

_____

_____

N.220   _The Chunky Carrot_   Yes / No

#dinner

green tea	¾ cup
carrot chunk	1
banana	1

HOW TO: boil the carrot until tender. Prepare the green tea. Place tea, carrot and banana in the blender and press START

TIPS: alternatively, juice the carrot, prepare only ½ cup of tea and blend all with the banana.

ADD YOUR COMMENT: _____

_____

_____

N.221 *Fruit Power* Yes / No

#lunch/dinner

peach	1
prune	1
banana	1
carrot	2
orange	½
ginger	15 ml
ice	4 cubes

HOW TO: juice carrot, orange and ginger. Blend everything together

TIPS: turn it in a smoothie bowl and top it with some chia seeds and flax seeds.

ADD YOUR COMMENT: _____
_____
_____

#lunch/dinner

fennel	½
cabbage	3 leaves
celery	1 stick
spinach	1 handful
cucumber	½
agave syrup	1 tsp
ice	half cup

HOW TO: juice the cucumber, celery and fennel. Place the juice in the blender and add the remaining ingredients. Press START

TIPS: here you have a healthy dinner that will help you to have a great night sleep

ADD YOUR COMMENT: _____
_____
_____

<u>Wasaaaabi</u>

#lunch

wasabi	1 tsp
avocado	1
carrot	4
agave syrup	1 tsp

HOW TO: juice the carrots and blend then all the ingredients together

TIPS: the wasabi is very spicy so if you are not use to it, add only the tip of a tsp to your blend. You can always add more later.

ADD YOUR COMMENT: _____
_____
_____

THE W@W FACTOR: *wasabi* or Japanese horseradish is a plant of the Brassicaceae family, which also includes horseradish and mustard. The plant grows naturally along stream beds in mountain river valleys in Japan.

A paste made from its ground rhizomes is used as a pungent condiment for sushi and other foods.

It is a rich source of fiber, protein, and energy. In terms of minerals, it contains calcium, iron, magnesium, phosphorus, potassium, sodium and zinc, which are all natural and necessary elements in our balanced diet. It is rich in vitamin C, thiamin, riboflavin, niacin, folate, vitamin A and vitamin B6. The plant also has high levels of certain antioxidants, like isothiocyanates, and it has zero cholesterol!

The health benefits of *wasabi* include providing a reduced risk of cancer and heart disease, as well as anti-inflammatory properties for joints and muscles. It also helps to defend against bacterial infections in the body and mouth, and can even reduce the irritating effects of seasonal allergies. This potent plant can be used to treat respiratory problems. *Wasabi*'s wealth of antioxidants helps to boost the immune system and remove harmful toxins from the body.

Wasabi can be a strong line of defense against certain respiratory tract pathogens. The gaseous component of wasabi, which causes such a powerful reaction in the nasal passages and sinuses, is actually the gaseous release of allyl isothiocyanate, which can actively inhibit the proliferation of respiratory tract pathogens like those that cause influenza and pneumonia. The smell and the sensation in your nose after eating it may be strong, but it can do a lot of good for your health and well-being.

N.224   *Cold Green*   *Yes / No*

#dessert

green tea	½ cup
dairy free vanilla ice cream	2 tbsp
kiwi	2
ice	4
banana	½

HOW TO: prepare the iced green tea and then place it in a blender with all the other ingredients. Press START

TIPS: add a tsp of spirulina for a greater body balance

ADD YOUR COMMENT: _____

_____

_____

N.225   *The Burning Passion*   *Yes / No*

#lunch

passion fruit	1
avocado	½
honey dew melon	1 slice
pineapple	1 slice
spirulina	1 tsp
wasabi	½ tsp
spinach	1 handful

HOW TO: juice the pineapple and the melon. Add all the ingredients listed above in the blender and press START

TIPS: great after a workout to burn few extra calories while filling your body with goodness.

ADD YOUR COMMENT: _____

_____

_____

The Twisted Lunch *Yes / No*

#lunch

sweet potato	½
coriander	3 leaves
cucumber	1
mango	½
nutmeg	a pinch
ice	4 cubes
ginger	15ml
spirulina	1 tsp

HOW TO: juice the cucumber and the ginger. Boil the sweet potato and run it under cold tap water. Blend then all together.

TIPS: add salt while boiling the sweet potato for extra flavour.

ADD YOUR COMMENT: _____

_____

_____

THE W@W FACTOR: *Coriander*, also known as **cilantro** or **Chinese parsley**, is an annual herb in the family Apiaceae. All parts of the plant are edible, but the fresh leaves and the dried seeds are the parts most traditionally used in cooking. *Coriander* is native to regions spanning from southern Europe and northern Africa to southwestern Asia.

As nutrients it includes high levels of dietary fiber, antioxidants, B vitamins, vitamin C, potassium, copper, magnesium, manganese, zinc, iron, and calcium. These seeds also provide a moderate amount of protein and fat, although they would need to be eaten in large quantities to have a notable effect on those intake levels. The smell of coriander comes from its antioxidants and volatile oils, which include linoleic acid, oleic acid, Linalool, alpha-pinene, and terpene, among others.

Cineole, one of the 11 components of the essential oils, and linoleic acid are both present in coriander, and they possess antirheumatic and antiarthritic properties. More specifically, they help reduce the swelling that is caused by these two conditions.

The health benefits of *coriander* includes its use in the treatment of skin inflammation; regulates cholesterol levels; ease diarrhea symptoms; helps with mouth ulcers; fights anemia, release indigestion, helps with menstrual disorders, fights smallpox, conjunctivitis, skin disorders, and blood sugar disorders, while also benefiting eye care.

Multiple studies have shown *coriander* to have strong anti-histamine properties that can reduce the uncomfortable effects of seasonal allergies and hay fever (rhinitis). Its oil can also be used to reduce allergic reactions that are caused due to contact with plants, insects, food, and other substances. Internally, it can ward off anaphylaxis, hives, and dangerous swelling of the throat and glands.

It's never a bad idea to protect yourself against allergic reactions, especially since it is difficult to know what you might be allergic to until you come in contact with it for the first time!

N.227   _The Super Berry_   Yes / No

#all times good

mandarin	2
strawberries	7
avocado	½
goji berries	1 tbsp
lemon	½

HOW TO: juice the lemon and the mandarin. Pour the juice in the blender and press START

TIPS: remember to peel the lime and mandarin before to put them in the juicer.

ADD YOUR COMMENT: _____

_____

_____

N.228   _The Bell Tomato_   Yes / No

#lunch

peanut butter	2 tbsp
tomato	1 large
green bell pepper	1
apple	1 ½
beetroot	1 ½

HOW TO: juice the apple and beetroot and pour the juice in the blender together with the other ingredients. Press START

TIPS: keep refrigerated for ~30 minutes before to drink

ADD YOUR COMMENT: _____

_____

_____

N.229   _Frozen Greeny_   Yes / No

          #lunch

green tea	¾ cup
dairy free vanilla ice cream	2 tbsp
spinach	1 handful
kale	1 handful
ice	3 cubes
avocado	½

HOW TO: prepare the tea in advance. Place all the ingredients in the blender and press START

TIPS: add also a tsp of spirulina powder for a more intense flavour

ADD YOUR COMMENT: _____

_____

_____

N.230   _Stardust_   Yes / No

          #breakfast

matcha	1 tsp
dates	2
soy yoghurt	3 tbsp
ice	4 cubes
carrot	3 large

HOW TO: juice the carrots. Place all the ingredients in the blender and press START

TIPS: use coconut yoghurt instead of the soy one for a more complex texture.

ADD YOUR COMMENT: _____

_____

_____

N.231   *The Greatest Night*   Yes / No
#lunch

mango	½
lime	½
soy yoghurt	2 tbsp
kale	1 handful
mix seeds	1 flat tbsp
ginger	15 ml
beetroot	2
apple	½

HOW TO: juice the beetroot, lime and apple. Blend all the ingredients together.

TIPS: as mix seed use a mix of chia, flax, pumpkin, hemp, sunflower seeds

ADD YOUR COMMENT: _____
_____
_____

N.232   *a mindset*   Yes / No
#dinner

apple	2 ½
banana	2
wasabi	½ tsp
pear	1 small

HOW TO: juice the apple. Blend all the ingredients together.

TIPS: add 4 ice cubes in the smoothie glass

ADD YOUR COMMENT: _____
_____
_____

Oham   Yes / No
                #dinner

camomile tea	½ cup
passion fruit	1
mango	½
mint	3 leaves
apple chunk	⅓
strawberries	2

HOW TO: prepare the tea in advance. Place all the ingredients in the blender and press START

TIPS: add few ice cubes in your smoothie glass

ADD YOUR COMMENT: _____
_____
_____

Kiss Me   Yes / No

#dinner

mint tea	¾ cup
mint leaves	3 leaves
ginger	15 ml
carrot chunk	1
mango chunk	½

HOW TO: prepare the mint tea in advance. Juice the ginger. Boil the carrot until tender. Place all the ingredients in the blender and press START

TIPS: in order to prepare the mint tea, you can either use the tea bag or leave mint leaves in infusion and let the water cool down (takes longer). If you leave the mint leaves in infusion you may also great 1 piece of ginger and let it boil together. In this way you can avoid to use the juicer and you will have less equipment to wash (real important!)

ADD YOUR COMMENT: _____

_____

_____

N.235   *A surprise taste*   Yes / No

#lunch/dinner

grapefruit	1
figs	2
kiwi	2
strawberries	6
agave syrup	1 tsp
grapes	6

HOW TO: juice the grapefruit and the kiwis. Add all the ingredients to the blender and press START

TIPS: remember to peel the grapefruit and the kiwis before to place it in the blender. Add one extra tsp of agave syrup if you wish for extra sweetness.

ADD YOUR COMMENT: _____

_____

_____

N.236   *Pick a cherry*   Yes / No

#dinner

mandarin	2
cherry	8 pitted
peach	1
apple	1

HOW TO: juice apple and mandarin. Pit the cherries and chop the peach. Blend all the ingredients together.

TIPS: this is a tasty and refreshing snack. Carry it with you for a energising break at work.

ADD YOUR COMMENT: _____

_____

_____

<u>Hempfullness</u>

#lunch

sweet potato	½
zucchini	½
black pepper	a pinch
hemp milk	¾ cup
salt	a pinch
apple chunk	½

HOW TO: boil sweet potato and the courgette until tender. Chop the apple and place all the ingredients in the blender. Press START.

TIPS: add already a bit of salt in the boiling water, blend it all together and then decide for yourself if you need an extra pinch of salt.

My advice is to make this a smoothie bowl: perfect either for lunch that for dinner and top it with some mix seeds.

ADD YOUR COMMENT: _____

_____

_____

THE W@W FACTOR: *Zucchini* or **courgette** is a summer squash which can reach nearly 1 metre in length, but is usually harvested when still immature at about 15 to 25 cm. *Zucchini* has its origin in America and is available in yellow, light green, and dark green color. Today, the largest producers of this squash include Japan, China, Romania, Italy, Turkey, Egypt, and Argentina. It is grown year-round and can be eaten raw, sliced or in cooked form. Even though zucchini is a fruit, it is usually cooked as a vegetable because it is best when eaten in cooked dishes. If you are looking for a way to lose weight in a healthy way, it's time for you to learn about the health benefits of zucchini. *Zucchini* is well-known to reduce weight, yet boost the nutrient value of your diet. Moreover, it helps enhance vision and prevent all the diseases that occur from vitamin C deficiency like scurvy, sclerosis, and easy bruising. It helps cure asthma, protect cardiovascular system and gives relief from aching symptoms and rheumatoid arthritis.Already being an outstanding source of manganese and vitamin C, *zucchini* is also the best source of dietary fiber that will keep your body in the best shape for the long run. It also contains vitamin A, magnesium, folate, potassium, copper, and phosphorus. This summer squash also has a high content of omega-3 fatty acids, zinc, niacin, and protein. Moreover, vitamin B1, vitamin B6, vitamin B2, and calcium in zucchini assure optimal health. It is probably the best squash having an array of nutrients, including sugar, carbohydrates, soluble and insoluble fiber, sodium, minerals, amino acids, and more. The folate ingredient of this squash is highly recommended for pregnant women as well.

N.238   *Cranberry mania*   Yes / No

#breakfast/lunch

flaxseeds	1 tsp
figs	2
dairy free vanilla ice cream	2 tbsp
banana	1
hemp milk	¾ cup
blueberries	1 handful
cranberries	1 handful

HOW TO: place all the ingredients in the blender and press START.

TIPS: is an amazing blend to pour in a cup and scoop your way until the end

ADD YOUR COMMENT: _____

_____

_____

N.239   *Lemon Cake*   Yes / No

#dessert

poppy seed	1 tsp
lemon juice	½
lemon zest	1
crumbled pound cake	½ cup
agave syrup	1 tsp
hemp milk	¾ cup

HOW TO: place all the ingredients in the blender and press START

TIPS: there is not need to use a juicer for the lemon but simply squeeze it straight inside the blender.

ADD YOUR COMMENT: _____

_____

_____

N.240   *Lemon Butter*   Yes / No

#breakfast/lunch

almond butter	1 tbsp
lemon	½
strawberry	5
cherry	5
cucumber	1

HOW TO: place all the ingredients in the blender. Squeeze half lemon inside the blender. Press START

TIPS: add few ice cubes or keep it in the fridge for around 30 minutes before to drink.

ADD YOUR COMMENT: _____

_____

_____

N.241   *Explosion of Sweetness*   Yes / No

#snack/dinner

wasabi	½ tsp
watermelon	¾ cup
pineapple	½ cup

HOW TO: juice the watermelon until your smoothie cup is almost full. Chop the pineapple until half of your cup is full. Blend all together.

TIPS: add few ice cubes in your blender for a creamier texture

ADD YOUR COMMENT: _____

_____

_____

Pudding Mania

#lunch

rice pudding	½ cup
potato	1 small
avocado	½
rice milk	½ cup
agave syrup	1 tsp
turmeric	1 tsp

HOW TO: prepare the pudding in advance. Boil the potato in advance. Add all the ingredients, once ready, in the blender and press START

TIPS: to prepare the pudding, cook the rice and, when almost ready, take the water out and let it slow cook with rice or soy milk and 1 tsp of sugar.

ADD YOUR COMMENT: _____
_____
_____

THE W@W FACTOR: *Rice* is the seed of the grass species Oryza Sativa (Asian Rice) and Oryza glaberrima (African rice). As a cereal grain, is the most widely consumed staple food in the world, especially in Asia. The grain comes in more than 40,000 varieties with different shapes, sizes, texture, aroma, and colors. Different types of *rice* include white, brown, rose, noodle, black pearl, red yeast, wild, jasmine, and sushi rice, among others. They can be long grain, medium grain, and short grain and take a very short preparation time. Most varieties contain a high amount of carbohydrates and protein. The fiber content varies according to types of *rice*. For eg., brown rice has more fiber than white rice and therefore, is a healthy option. It is also rich in minerals like calcium, iron, magnesium, phosphorus, potassium, manganese, selenium, and copper. The vitamins in it include niacin, pantothenic acid, and thiamine. It is a great food for people wanting a gluten-free option and it contains negligible fat.
Since *rice* is abundant in carbohydrates, it acts as fuel for the body and aids in the normal functioning of the brain. Low levels of fat, cholesterol, and sodium also help reduce obesity and associated conditions. It is also involved in prevent cancer, help with skin care, improve metabolism, boost cardiovascular health, it has diuretic and digestive qualities and aid in control the blood pressure.

The Long List Yes / No

#lunch

fruit of the forest	1 handful
mango	½
avocado	½
cucumber	1
parsley	3 leaves
ginger	15 ml
lime	½
wasabi	½ tsp

HOW TO: juice ginger, cucumber and lime. Chop and place the rest of the ingredients in the blender and mix all together.

TIPS: perfect for lunch or dinner. pour it in a bowl and top it with your daily dose of flax seeds (1 tsp sprinkled on the bowl).

ADD YOUR COMMENT: _____

_____

_____

N.244   *The Dark Berry*   Yes / No
#dinner

cranberries	1 flat tbsp
beetroot	2
celery	2 stalks
raspberries	1 handful

HOW TO: juice beetroot and celery and blend all together with the berries.

TIPS: add 3 ice cubes in the glass and stir 1 tsp of spirulina if you like

ADD YOUR COMMENT: _____

_____

_____

N.245   *What a Day!*   Yes / No
#all day good

figs	2
almond butter	1 tbsp
carrot	3 large
mango	1

HOW TO: juice only the carrots. Place all the ingredients in the blender and press START.

TIPS: it depend of the size of your cup, you may need extra juice. If this is the case, add extra cucumber juice so that also the flavour is not too strong.

ADD YOUR COMMENT: _____

_____

_____

N.246   _The wedding Wish_   _Yes / No_

#all day good

mandarin	1
fig	2
apple	2
avocado	½
passion fruit	1
coriander	4 leaves

HOW TO: juice the apple and avocado. Place all the ingredients in the blender and press START.

TIPS: pour it in a bowl and top it with chia seeds and fig slice.

ADD YOUR COMMENT: _____

_____

_____

N.247   _The Genie in the Bottle_   _Yes / No_

#dessert

amarena cherry syrup	1 tsp
carrot	3 large
spinach	1 handful
figs	1
banana	½
raspberries	1 handful
maple syrup	1 tsp

HOW TO: juice only the carrots and then add the juice to the blender together with the other ingredients. Press START

TIPS: ideal either for lunch that for dinner. Take it with you at work! Your skin will thank you.

ADD YOUR COMMENT: _____

_____

_____

N.248   _The Brown we Like_   Yes / No
#breakfast/lunch

lemon	½
avocado	1
chocolate shavings	1 tbsp
cocoa	1 tsp
apple juice	2 ½
figs	1

HOW TO: juice the apple and the lemon. Place all the ingredients in the blender and press START

TIPS: keep it refrigerated!

ADD YOUR COMMENT: _____
_____
_____

N.249   _Over the Moon_   Yes / No
#lunch

rocket	4 leaves
beetroot	2
chickpeas	1 tbsp
peanut butter	1 tbsp
banana	½
spirulina	1 tsp
water as needed	

HOW TO: juice the beetroot only. Add all the ingredients in the blender and press START.

TIPS: add as much water as you need to feel your cup of smoothie

ADD YOUR COMMENT: _____
_____
_____

#lunch

soaked cashew nuts	1 tbsp
chickpeas	1 tbsp
cantaloup melon	¾ cup of juice
avocado	½

HOW TO: juice enough melon to fill your smoothie cup. Mix all the ingredients together.

TIPS: if you find the taste of the melon too much for you, juice only ⅓ of the cup and add plain water

ADD YOUR COMMENT: _____

_____

_____

Veggie Mania Plus *Yes / No*

#**lunch**

chickpeas	1 tbsp
broccoli	½ cup
tomato	1 large
carrot	2 large
apple	1
radish	1

HOW TO: juice the carrot and the apple. Add all the other ingredients in the blender and press START

TIPS: use pre-cooked chickpeas or cook it yourself. Use only the top tender part of the broccoli for this smoothie.

ADD YOUR COMMENT: _____

_____

_____

THE W@W FACTOR: *Radish* is an edible root vegetable of the Brassicaceae family, domesticated in Europe in pre-Roman times. Nowaday, *radish* are cultivated and consumed worldwide, mostly eaten raw as part of a crunchy salad. There are numerous varieties, changing in size, flavor, colour, and length of time they take to mature.

From a nutritional point of view, *radish* is rich in vitamin and mineral containing vitamin C, E, A, K potassium, folic acid, phosphorus, zinc, magnesium, copper, iron, calcium, manganese, fiber and vitamin B-complex. It is also very high in antioxidant.

Radish is very good for the liver and the stomach acting as a powerful detoxifier: it facilitates digestion, water retention and eliminates constipation. *Radish* are diuretic in nature which means that they increase the production of urine.

Radishes are very filling, which mean that they satisfy your hunger without running up the calorie count. They are also low in digestible carbohydrates, high in roughage, and contain a lot of water, thus becoming a very good dietary option for those who are determined to lose weight. Furthermore, they are high in fiber and low on the glycemic index, which means that they increase regular bowel movements, which helps in weight loss, and increases the efficiency of metabolism for all bodily processes.

Radish are a great source of anthocyanins, a type of flavonoids, that reduces the chances of cardiovascular diseases and they have anti-cancer and anti-inflammatory properties. Radishes are an anti-congestive, meaning that they decrease congestion of the respiratory system including irritation of the nose, throat, windpipe, and lungs that can come from colds, infections, allergies, and other causes.

In general, *radish* is involved in lower blood pressure, control diabetes, maintain a natural moist skin, protect kidney, liver and gallbladder and boost immunity.

N.252   *No Border*   Yes / No
                    #dinner

liquorice	½ stalk
banana	1
carrot	4 large
passion fruit	1

HOW TO: juice only the carrot. Add all the other ingredients in the blender and press START

TIPS: add few ice cubes in the glass

ADD YOUR COMMENT: _____

_____

_____

Never Without! *Yes / No*

#breakfast

vanilla flavour	3 drops
strawberry	5
soy yoghurt	2 tbsp
hemp milk	¾ cup
pear	2 small

HOW TO: wash carefully strawberries and pear. Dice the pears. Add all the ingredients in the above list inside the blender. Press START

TIPS: add a protein powder of you choice. This smoothie is a great breakfast option. With a cup of plain coffee (opt only for americano or espresso) next to it is all you can wish for.

ADD YOUR COMMENT: _____

_____

_____

<u>*Hard Awakening*</u>   *Yes / No*

#breakfast

peanut butter	1 tbsp
liquorice	½ stalks
almond milk	¾ cup
banana	1
ground almond	1 tbsp

HOW TO: prepare all your ingredients and add it in the blender. Press START.

TIPS: use ripe banana when smoothing. It gives a less bitter but creamier taste

ADD YOUR COMMENT: _____

_____

_____

THE W@W FACTOR: *liquorice* plant is an herbaceous perennial legume native to southern Europe and part of Asia. *Liquorice* extract are either used as candy or sweetener that as part of herbalism and traditional medicine. The eaten *liquorice* is the root of the Glycyrrhiza glabra plant.

From a nutritional point of view *liquorice* contains vitamin B, manganese and phosphorus, essential oils, sugar and starch, phytoestrogen, gums, amino acid, flavonoids, and glycyrrhizic acid as one of the main active constituent.

Liquorice or licorice helps the digestive system by soothing gastric and abdominal disorder including stomach ulcers, heartburn and other inflammation issues. Provide respiratory relief by reducing symptoms of cold and flu such as cough and sore throat. Promote skin health by reducing the presence of dermatitis, cysts and eczema. It also helps to keep the blood pressure under control.

Furthermore, it is used as remedy to reduce the amount of stress experienced in the everyday life.

Round and Round

#lunch

fennel	½
potato	1 small
turmeric	1 tsp
linseed	1 tsp
tomato	1 large
apple	1
cucumber	¾

HOW TO: juice the apple and the cucumber. boil the potato until tender. When ready, place all the ingredients in the blender and press START

TIPS: there is a lot of heat in this blend...add few ice cubes straight in the mixer or keep your smoothie refrigerated.

ADD YOUR COMMENT: _____

_____

_____

THE W@W FACTOR: *Potato* is a starchy, tuberous crop introduced to Europe in the second half of the 16th century by the Spanish. Over 99% of the presently cultivated *potatoes* descended from a variety firstly originated in south-central Chile. There are now over a thousand of different kind of potatoes.

Nowadays, *potatoes* are one of the most common and important food sources on the planet with a wealth of health benefits and nutritional value that makes it essential as a staple dietary item. Potatoes are rich in potassium. The concentration is highest in the skin and just beneath it; therefore is beneficial to eat the potatoes with the skin still on. They also contains calcium, iron and phosphorus. *Potatoes* contains a large amount of vitamin C, but they also have vitamin A, vitamin B and vitamin P (phytonutrients). Surprisingly, 70-80% of potatoes weight is due to their water content. And they contains around 17% of starch and are probably the best source of it.

Potatoes are primarily made of carbohydrates and very little protein which makes it ideal for gain healthy weight and it makes it also very easy to digest. Plus, it supports skin health, reduces inflammation, lowers blood pressure, increases brain function, treat kidney stone and lowers the risk of heart diseases and cancer.

N.256   *<u>Sparkling Moments</u>*   *Yes / No*

#lunch/dinner

sparkling water	¾ cup
strawberry	4
mango	½
papaya	½
cucumber	⅓
celery	1 stalk
pinch of black pepper	

HOW TO: use only the blender! Wash, chop and blend all the fruits and vegetables in the ingredient list above.

TIPS: if you don't like have water in your smoothie, change it! juice the cucumber and celery instead.

ADD YOUR COMMENT: _____

_____

_____

N.257   *<u>The Tiger Within</u>*   *Yes / No*

#lunch

celery	3 stalks
cherry	5
cantaloup melon	1 slice
banana	1
spinach	1 handful
spirulina	1 tsp

HOW TO: Juice celery and melon. Remove the kernel from the cherries. Add all the ingredients in the blender and press START

TIPS: don't waste food! use the vegetables you have already in your fridge: instead of spinach you could opt for kale or broccoli.

ADD YOUR COMMENT: _____

_____

_____

N.258   <u>A walk in the sun</u>   Ye<i>s</i> / N<i>o</i>
            #dinner

turmeric   1 tsp
carrot   3 large
papaya   1

HOW TO: juice the carrots and add the juice to the blender together with the chopped papaya and the tsp of turmeric powder

TIPS: if you have fresh turmeric in your fridge, don't worry about buying the powder. Grate your turmeric straight in the blender. Enjoy!

ADD YOUR COMMENT: _____
_____
_____

N.259   <u>Fire Up</u>   Ye<i>s</i> / N<i>o</i>
                       #dinner

dragon fruit   ½ cup
banana   1
mint   2 leaves
cinnamon   1 tsp
pineapple   ¾ cup of juice

HOW TO: juice the pineapple only. Mix all the ingredients together in your blender and press START.

TIPS: add a tsp of acai berry powder to increase the energetic power of your drink...and is good on your skin too!

ADD YOUR COMMENT: _____
_____
_____

N.260   *Cake time!*   Yes / No

#dessert

crumbled pound cake	½ cup
mango	1
choco chip	1 tbsp
coconut milk	¾ cup

HOW TO: blend all the ingredients together

TIPS: if you don't have chocolate chips available, simple cacao is a great alternative

ADD YOUR COMMENT: _____

_____

_____

N.261   *The King of The Land*   Yes / No

#lunch

pumpkin	½ cup
fig	2
spinach	1 handful
pear	1
carrot	3 large

HOW TO: juice the carrot. Chop the other ingredients and mix them all in the blender. Press START

TIPS: a teaspoon of wheatgrass will make the difference...try it out!

ADD YOUR COMMENT: _____

_____

_____

N.262 *Ciao Chai* Yes / No
#snack/dinner

chai tea	¾ cup
cinnamon	1 tsp
blueberry	2 handful
kiwi	2

HOW TO: prepare the tea in advance....make it iced!
Place all the ingredients in the blender and press START

TIPS: if you like only thick smoothies add one banana
to your blend.

ADD YOUR COMMENT: _____
_____
_____

N.263 *Radiant Skin* Yes / No
#all times good

orange	2
acai	1 tbsp
mango	1
ginger	15 ml

HOW TO: juice orange and ginger and add all the ingredients
in the blender to smooth.

TIPS: you can either use the acai powder (1 tbsp) or frozen acai
(1 cube)

ADD YOUR COMMENT: _____
_____
_____

<u>Kale this Passion</u>

#all times good

pomegranate	1 tbsp
kale	1 handful
cucumber	1
mix berry	1 handful

HOW TO: juice the cucumber. Add all the ingredients in the blender and press START

TIPS: peel the pomegranate and prepare a cup with all the content. Store it in the fridge and enjoy as snack on is own, in a smoothie or juice it for a refreshing drink.

ADD YOUR COMMENT: _____

_____

_____

THE W@W FACTOR: *Pomegranate* is a fruit-bearing small tree, growing 5 to 10m high, has multiple spiny branches. The flower are bright red, as the fruit, with three to seven petals. It has been cultivated since ancient times throughout the Mediterranean regions. Right now, India is the world's largest producer of pomegranate.

Pomegranate seeds get their vibrant red hue from polyphenol which are powerful antioxidants which can help remove free radicals, protect cells from damage and remove inflammation.

They also contains antiviral and antitumor properties together with vitamins A, C and E and folic acid as well as calcium, potassium and iron. Flavonols in *pomegranate* juice may help block the inflammation that contributes to osteoarthritis and cartilage damage. It protect heart and arteries by reducing cholesterol and blood pressure. Improve learning and memories.

Pomegranate juice may be the new sport performance enhancer: it may help reduce soreness and improve strength recovery and it also decreases oxidative damage caused by exercise.

The Best is Simple Yes / No

#snack/dinner

pear	2
peach	2
apple	1 ½
carrot	2 large

HOW TO: juice the apple and carrot and add the juice in the blender with the chop peach and pear. Press START

TIPS: I believe this smoothie is perfect in it's simple version but if you like add a spicy of your favourites (ginger, turmeric and so on)

ADD YOUR COMMENT: _____
_____
_____

A full Day

#breakfast

poppy seeds	1 flat tbsp
almond butter	1 tbsp
golden syrup	1 tsp
cinnamon	1 tsp
soy milk	¾ cup

HOW TO: place all the ingredients in the blender and press START

TIPS: this is not a very creamy blend. If you desire extra thickness include also a banana in your mix.

ADD YOUR COMMENT: _____

_____

_____

THE W@W FACTOR: *Golden Syrup* or light treacle is a thick, amber-coloured form of inverted sugar syrup made of the process of refining sugar cane into sugar. It is used in a variety of baking recipes and it is used by many vegans as a honey substitute. Created by Charles Eastick, an English chemist, in 1883, was first canned and sold in 1885. In 2006 it was recognised by Guinness World Records has having the world's oldest branding and packaging.

N.267   _The Space Shuttle_   Yes / No
         #breakfast/lunch

rocket	4 leaves
blueberries	2 handful
agave syrup	1 tsp
coconut yoghurt	3 tbsp
coconut milk	¾ cup

HOW TO: wash carefully rockets and blueberries. Place all the ingredients in the blender and press START

TIPS: if you find rocket to have a too strong of a flavour for you, swap it with kale or spinach

ADD YOUR COMMENT: _____
_____
_____

N.268   _Olive Land_   Yes / No
         #lunch

beetroot	2
green olives	5
rocket	3 leaves
figs	2
ice	½ cup
salt	a pinch

HOW TO: juice only the beetroot. Place then all the ingredient in the blender and press START.

TIPS: if you don't want use ice, add instead plain water for ½ a cup

ADD YOUR COMMENT: _____
_____
_____

An Explosive Day

#breakfast

granola	2 tbsp
oat flakes	1 tbsp
ground almond	1 flat tbsp
peanut butter	1 tbsp
almond milk	¾ cup
coffee powder	1 tsp
maple syrup	1 tsp
fig	1
spinach	1 handful

HOW TO: simply organise your ingredients and place it in your blender. Press START

TIPS: make it your morning smoothie bowl. Place it in a bowl and top it with little extra granola, oats and peanut butter. Take a picture now! your INSTAGRAM feed will thank you

ADD YOUR COMMENT: _____

_____

_____

Food of the Gods   Yes / No

#lunch

acai berry (frozen or powder)	1 tbsp
zucchini	⅓
celery	2 stalks
banana	1
cucumber	1
ginger	15 ml

HOW TO: place the zucchini in boiling water and cook it very well. In the meanwhile, juice the celery, cucumber and ginger. Add all the ingredients in the blender and press START

TIPS: add also few ice cubes in the blender or store it in the fridge

ADD YOUR COMMENT: _____

_____

_____

The Alien on Earth

#lunch

aubergine	3 small cubes
avocado	½
fennel	½
apple	2
carrot	2
red paprika powder	1 tsp

HOW TO: juice apple and carrot. Boil the aubergine until very well cooked and run it under cold water. Place all the ingredients in the blender and press START

TIPS: refrigerate it for around 30 minutes before to drink

ADD YOUR COMMENT: _____

_____

_____

THE W@W FACTOR: *Aubergine* or eggplant, is a species of nightshade grown for its edible fruit. The flower is white to purple, with a five-lobed corolla and yellow stamens. The egg-shaped, glossy, purple fruit has white flesh with a meaty texture, that quickly turns brown when cut open. It has been cultivated in Southern and Eastern Asia since prehistory.

Aubergine are an excellent source of dietary fiber. They are also a great source of vitamin B1, B6 and potassium, copper, magnesium and manganese. They are also rich in antioxidants, especially nasunin, found in the aubergine skin and that gives it the purple colour.

Within the health benefits of *eggplant* we find: helps digestion and weight loss thanks to the high amount of fiber contained in it; prevent cancer thanks to the antioxidant property that fight against free radicals; have antiviral and antibacterial qualities; improve bone health thanks to the iron and calcium; prevent anemia; improve brain function thanks to the phytonutrients found in the eggplant in high levels; improve heart health and manage diabetes.

N.272   *Warm under the Shade*   *Yes / No*

#lunch

coriander	3 leaves
papaya	1
honey dew melon	¾ cup of juice
ginger	15 ml
ice	3 cubes
turmeric	1 tsp

HOW TO: juice only the melon. Place all the other ingredients in the blender and press START

TIPS: this blend has a lot of spice in it. Feel free to modify the amount of ginger, turmeric and coriander respecting your habit and your needs.

ADD YOUR COMMENT: _____

_____

_____

N.273   *Back to Basic*   *Yes / No*

#breakfast/lunch

dragon fruit	½ cup
basil	2 leaves
almond	1 handful
almond milk	½ cup
papaya	½ cup

HOW TO: wash, chop and place your ingredients in the blender. Press START

TIPS: is nice to drink for a afternoon snack or dinner time. Enjoy!

ADD YOUR COMMENT: _____

_____

_____

N.274   _Never without you_   Yes / No
#lunch/dinner

carrot	2 large
radish	1
kiwi	1
beetroot	1
coriander	2 leaves
fennel	½

HOW TO: juice the carrots and beetroot and blend then all the ingredients together.

TIPS: you can either juice the fennel or blend it with the rest

ADD YOUR COMMENT: _____

_____

_____

N.275   _Extra Berry_   Yes / No
#dinner

mix berry	2 tbsp
ice	3 cubes
agave syrup	1 tsp
spinach	1 handful
watermelon	¾ cup

HOW TO: juice the watermelon until filling ¾ of your cup. Pour the juice in the blender and add the other ingredients.

TIPS: add a tsp of acai powder for extra berry benefits on your body

ADD YOUR COMMENT: _____

_____

_____

N.276   _Shining Armour_   Yes / No

#dinner

mango juice	¾ cup
ginger	15 ml
ice	½ cup
banana	1 ½

HOW TO: juice enough mango to fill up ¾ of your smoothie cup. Juice the ginger (or grate it). place all the ingredients in the blender and press START

TIPS: option to chop half mango and use water base for a faster result

ADD YOUR COMMENT: _____

_____

_____

N.277   _In the end of the tunnel_   Yes / No

#lunch

beetroot	1
cucumber	1
banana	1
ginger zest	as needed

HOW TO: juice only the cucumber. place all the ingredients in the blender and press START

TIPS: add few ice cubes in your smoothie glass

ADD YOUR COMMENT: _____

_____

_____

N.278 *Out of my Chest* *Yes / No*

#breakfast

chestnut	3
soy milk	¾ cup
soy yoghurt	2 tbsp
passion fruit	1
ice	4 cubes

HOW TO: prepare your ingredients then blend it all together

TIPS: which dairy free milk do you have today in your fridge? no need to buy many different type but simply use what you already have

ADD YOUR COMMENT: _____

_____

_____

N.279 *The Health Solution* *Yes / No*

#lunch

celery	2 stalks
zucchini	½
banana	1
lime zest	1
ice	½ cup
beetroot	2

HOW TO: cook the zucchini in advance until well cooked. Place all the ingredients in the blender together with the juice of the celery and beetroot and press START

TIPS: if you need extra liquid base use plain water

ADD YOUR COMMENT: _____

_____

_____

N.280   _Taste of Summer_   _Yes / No_

#dinner

aloe vera	¾ cup
mango	1
spinach	1 handful

HOW TO: place in the blender all the ingredients and press START.

TIPS: I use aloe vera juice easy to find in any shop!

ADD YOUR COMMENT: _____

_____

_____

N.281   _Mind the Gap!_   _Yes / No_

#breakfast

cherry	2 handful
coconut yoghurt	3 tbsp
coconut cream	1 tbsp
mango	½
banana	1
coconut milk	½ cup

HOW TO: pit the cherries. place all the other ingredients in the blender and press START

TIPS: the coconut cream I use is the fat part of the canned coconut milk. Keep it in the fridge overnight before to use it!

ADD YOUR COMMENT: _____

_____

_____

N.282   *Sweet taste*   Yes / No

#dessert

soy custard cream	2 tbsp
amarena cherry	1 handful
banana	1
raspberry	1 handful
ice	½ cup
soy milk	⅓ of the cup

HOW TO: place all the ingredients in the blender and press START.

TIPS: any other alternative of plant base custard cream you have available will be perfectly fine.

ADD YOUR COMMENT: _____

_____

_____

N.283   *Lunch is served*   Yes / No

#lunch

orange	1
mandarin	2
avocado	1
lime zest	½
lemon zest	½
cherries	1 handful

HOW TO: juice the orange and the mandarin. Grate the lime and lemon straight in the blender. Pit the cherries. Place all the ingredients in the blender and press START

TIPS: rich in flavour, is perfect for detox and energize your body at the same time

ADD YOUR COMMENT: _____

_____

_____

N.284   *Purple fashion*   Yes / No

#lunch/dinner

beetroot	1
blueberry	2 handful
ginger	15 ml
cherry	2 handful
apple	1

HOW TO: juice the apple, ginger and beetroot. Pit the cherries and blend all the ingredients together

TIPS: if you don't have a juicer. Place the blueberries in the blender, pit the cherries and add them together. Zest the ginger straight in the blender. Chop and add the beetroot. Chop ¼ of the apple and add it to the blend. Add ½ cup of plain water

ADD YOUR COMMENT: _____

_____

_____

N.285   *Ginger Love*   Yes / No

#breakfast

chia seed	1 flat tbsp
turmeric	1 tsp
ginger zest	1 tsp
strawberry	4
oat flakes	1 tbsp
banana	1
water	½ cup
ice	½ cup

HOW TO: you only need the blender! Place all the ingredients together and press START

TIPS: is perfect for every meal. Enjoy it as a breakfast, lunch or dinner alternative.

ADD YOUR COMMENT: _____

_____

_____

Sexy Softness   Yes / No
                    #dessert

lavender tea	¾ cup
amarena cherry	1 handful
banana	1
agave syrup	1 tsp
ice	½ cup
raspberries	1 handful

HOW TO: prepare the tea in advance. Let it cool down. Add all the ingredients to the blender and press START

TIPS: perfect to share with your loved one after a romantic dinner. Pour it in a fancy glass and top it with extra cherries.

ADD YOUR COMMENT: _____
_____
_____

Great for Health   Yes / No

#dinner

orange zest	of ½ orange
cucumber juice	¾ cup
ginger zest	1 tsp
kale	1 handful
ice	6 cubes

HOW TO: grate the skin of ½ orange and a little ginger. Juice the cucumber only. Wash the kale properly and add it to the mix. Press START

TIPS: if you don't have a juicer, chop half cucumber and place it in the blender. Add ½ cup of water

ADD YOUR COMMENT: _____

_____

_____

Cleansed and Charged

#lunch

romaine lettuce	1 handful
avocado	1
cilantro	2 leaves
apple	1
carrot	2 large
ginger	15 ml
ginger zest	1 tsp

HOW TO: juice apple, carrot and ginger. Add the juice in the blender. Peel and add the avocado. Grate the ginger and add it to the mix. Wash carefully lettuce and cilantro and mix all together. Press START

TIPS: juicer free solution. Add an extra tsp of ginger zest instead of the juice. Add ¼ of chopped apple and ½ chopped carrot (it depends of the strength of your blender, you may need to boil the carrot first to make it tender). Add ½ cup of water.

ADD YOUR COMMENT: _____

_____

_____

The Sweet Grapefruit   *Yes / No*

#breakfast

granola	2 tbsp
grapefruit	1
mango	1
agave syrup	2 tsp
ice	½ cup
soy yoghurt	3 tbsp

HOW TO: juice the grapefruit and pour the juice in your blender. Add then granola, ice, yoghurt and syrup. Peel and chop the mango and add it to the mix. Press START

TIPS: if you don't have a juicer, proceed in exactly the same way. Instead of juice the grapefruit, simply take the skin out and chop it. Grapefruit has a high content of water and it will turn liquid very quickly in your blender too. Only make sure that the grapefruit is the closest thing to the blades in your blender. Add little water if required.

ADD YOUR COMMENT: _____

_____

_____

<u>*Waltz of the Veggies*</u> Yes / No

#lunch

green olives	4
cabbage	2 leaves
peanut butter	2 tbsp
soy yoghurt	2 tbsp
carrot	3 large
celery	1 stalk

HOW TO: juice the carrots. Pour the juice in your blender. Add the olives, the peanut butter and the yoghurt. Wash and chop the celery stick and the cabbage. Add the vegetables to the mix and press START

TIPS: if you don't have a juicer. Chop and boil one large carrot until tender. Run it under cold water and then place it in your blender. Add ½ cup of plain water or ½ cup of soy milk and blend

ADD YOUR COMMENT: _____

_____

_____

Classic Tenderness   Yes / No

#dinner

dates	2
banana	1
apple	2 ½
cranberry	1 tbsp
lime	½

HOW TO: juice the apples and the lime. Pour the juice in the blender and add the cranberries and the banana. Depit the dates and include it in the mix. Press START

TIPS: if you don't have a juicer. Cut a lime in half, remove the skin and place it in the blender. Wash and chope ¼ of a apple and place it in the blender. Add ½ cup of water before to blend.

ADD YOUR COMMENT: _____

_____

_____

N.292   *Mix Power*   Yes / No

#dinner

mango	1
kale	1 handful
sparkling water	¾ cup
ice	4 cubes

HOW TO: you only need the blender. wash the kale thoroughly and place it in the blender together with the ice and water. Peel and chop the mango and add it to the mix. Press START

TIPS: drink it either as a snack or as a light dinner. Cheers!

ADD YOUR COMMENT: _____

_____

_____

N.293 _Leaf of Life_ Yes / No

#dinner

mix leaves	2 handful
lemon	½
pear	1 large
fig	2
cucumber	¾ of a cup

HOW TO: juice the cucumber until having your cup ¾ full. Pour the juice in the blender. Squeeze the ½ lemon straight into the blender. Wash the mix salad. Wash and chop pear and fig. Join the ingredients together and press START

TIPS: if you don't have a juicer, then chop ⅓ of the cucumber and add it to the mix. Fill with ½ cup of water and press START

ADD YOUR COMMENT: _____
_____
_____

Colours of Nature

#lunch

apricot	1
romaine lettuce	1 handful
avocado	½
banana	½
ginger	20 ml
ice	½ cup
carrot	2 large

HOW TO: juice carrot and ginger. Pour the juice in the blender. Add the banana and the avocado. Wash and chop the apricot. Wash and chop the lettuce. Add it to your mix and press START

TIPS: if you don't have a juicer chop half carrot for your mix (you may need to boil the carrot if your blender doesn't have a high speed). Add ½ cup of water or soy milk.

ADD YOUR COMMENT: _____

_____

_____

Silence in town   Yes / No

#breakfast

rice pudding	½ cup
lemon	½
kiwi	1
peach	2
rice milk	½ cup

HOW TO: prepare the rice pudding in advance. Let it cool down and then add it to the blender. Squeeze the lemon. Wash, peel and chop the kiwi. Wash and chop the peach. Add the rice milk and press START

TIPS: keep it refrigerating for around 30 minutes before to enjoy the mix.

ADD YOUR COMMENT: _____

_____

_____

Adagio

#dinner

mango	1
kiwi	2
dragon fruit	½
lime	½
ice	5 cubes

HOW TO: juice the mango, the lime and the kiwi. Pour the juice into the blender. Add the ice cubes and the chopped dragon fruit. Press START

TIPS: if you don't have a juicer, peel and chop the kiwis and add it to the mix. Peel and chop only 1 mango and add it to the mix. Add ½ cup of water or coconut milk and blend.

ADD YOUR COMMENT: _____

_____

_____

THE W@W FACTOR: *dragon fruit*, or pitaya fruit, is a fruit from Central America, South America, and Asia. It has a light sweet taste, an intense shape and color, and has a texture of between that of a kiwi and an apple.

In addition to being tasty and refreshing, *dragon fruit* contains a lot of water and other vital minerals with a variety of nutritional ingredients. It is rich in proteins, fiber, lycopene, and carbohydrates. It contains carotene, vitamin C, vitamin B, thiamine (vitamin B1), and riboflavin. The mineral wealth of this fruit includes calcium, phosphorus, iron, and sodium.

Dragon fruit is believed to contain phytonutrients that prevent various diseases. Also, there are polyunsaturated fatty acids like omega 3 and omega 6 fatty acids in the seeds of these fruits.

Dragon fruit has a number of health benefits including its ability to lower cholesterol, boost the immune system, prevent cancer, and heart disease, aid in weight loss, improve digestion, boost energy, defend against bacteria and fungi, and help in the overall functioning of the body's systems.

The Music I Create

#breakfast

spinach	2 handful
oat flakes	1 tbsp
chia seeds	1 flat tbsp
coconut peanut butter	2 tbsp
banana	1
soy milk	¾ cup

HOW TO: you only need the blender! place all the ingredients together and press START

TIPS: be careful! the chia seeds tend to stuck to the bottom, therefore is better if place it in between your ingredients. Also, if you don't find the coconut peanut butter it's okay, use the normal peanut butter and eventually swap for coconut milk instead of soy

ADD YOUR COMMENT: _____

_____

_____

The piano music

#lunch

spinach	1 handful
green olives	5
cherries	4
apple	2
celery	½ stalk
mint	2 leaves
basil	1 leave
ginger	15 ml

HOW TO: juice the apple and the celery with the ginger. Add the juice into the blender. Pit the cherries and the green olives. Wash properly spinach, mint and basil and blend all the ingredients together.

TIPS: if you don't have a juicer, chop the ½ celery and add it to the blend. Place ¼ of an apple chopped inside the blender too. Top with plain still water.

ADD YOUR COMMENT: _____

_____

_____

Wave away...   *Yes / No*

#dinner

lychee	4
basil	1 leave
kale	1 handful
peach	1
carrot	2
cucumber	½

HOW TO: juice the carrots and the cucumber. Pour the juice into the blender. Wash basil, kale and peach and add it to the mix. Use lychee in a can or peel the fresh one and add it to the mix. Press START

TIPS: if you don't have a juicer, chop ⅓ of the cucumber and add it to the mix. Chop 2 carrots cubes and add it to the mix. Top with water.

ADD YOUR COMMENT: _____

_____

_____

<u>When the Past comes by</u>   *Yes / No*

#**dinner**

basil	1 leave
radish	2
apple	1
cucumber	¾
lime	½

HOW TO: juice lime, cucumber and apple. Pour the juice in the blender. Wash basil and radish and add it to the mix. Press START

TIPS: if you don't have a juicer squeeze half of your lime straight in the blender, chop ½ of the cucumber and add it to the mix with one third of the apple. Top with water.

ADD YOUR COMMENT: _____

_____

_____

N.301   <u>Je t'Aime Comme ça</u>   *Yes / No*

#**lunch**

tomato	3 large
banana	1
ice	¾ of a cup
turmeric	1 tsp

HOW TO: wash the tomatoes and place it in the blender. Peel and add the banana. Add the rest of the ingredients and press START

TIPS: if you need bigger quantity add little water or an extra tomato. If you like it thicker add extra banana.

ADD YOUR COMMENT: _____

_____

_____

N.302   *La vita e' bella*   Yes / No

#lunch

onion	⅓
tomato	2 large
spinach	1 handful
cucumber	1
avocado	1
maple syrup	1 tsp

HOW TO: juice only the cucumber. Wash the tomato, chop it and remove the central part. Add all the ingredients to the blender and press START.

TIPS: if you don't have a juicer, add ½ of the cucumber chopped in the blender and add little water

ADD YOUR COMMENT: _____

_____

_____

N.303   *The Tan that stays*   Yes / No

#snack/dinner

carrot	2
kiwi	2
mango	½
ice	5 cubes

HOW TO: juice only the carrots. Peel kiwis and mango, chop it and place it in the blender. Add the ice cubes and the carrot juice and press START.

TIPS: if you aim for a refreshing juice, you can simply juice all the ingredients and add the ice cubes in your juice glass.

ADD YOUR COMMENT: _____

_____

_____

N.304   *Never Wrong*   Yes / No
#snack/dinner

carrot	2
kiwi	2
pineapple	⅓

HOW TO: juice the carrots. Peel the kiwis and add the fruit in the blender. Peel and chop the pineapple in small cubes and add it in the blender as well. Pour the carrot Juice in it and press START

TIPS: if you like, you can simply juice all the ingredients and have a refreshing snack.

ADD YOUR COMMENT: _____

_____

_____

N.305   *Green Supreme*   Yes / No
#lunch

pistachio	1 handful
avocado	1
kale	1 handful
apple	1
cucumber	¾
green pepper	½
flaxseed	1 tsp

HOW TO: juice apple and cucumber and pour then the juice in your blender. Add the rest of the ingredients and press START

TIPS: if you don't have a juicer, chop the cucumber in small cubes (⅓ of it) and add ½ cup of water

ADD YOUR COMMENT: _____

_____

_____

Vinyasa Flow   Yes / No

#lunch

butternut squash	½ cup
radish	2
cherry tomato	2
cauliflower	2 pieces
apple	1 ½
cucumber	½
celery	1 stalk

HOW TO: juice apple, cucumber and celery. Place the cauliflower and the butternut squash in boiling water so that will become tender. Wash and add the remaining ingredients in the blender. Press START

TIPS: if you don't have a juicer, chop the celery stick, ⅓ of cucumber and ¼ of the apple and add it to the blender with little water

ADD YOUR COMMENT: _____

_____

_____

<u>*A Turn of Page*</u>

#lunch

cabbage	½ cup
parsnip	⅓ cup
parsley	3 leaves
cherry tomato	4
beetroot	1
apple	2

HOW TO: juice the beetroot and the apples. Wash and chop the cabbage and the parsnip. Wash the cherry tomatoes and the parsley. Add all the ingredients in your blender and press START

TIPS: if you don't have a juicer, chop the beetroot and add it to the mix. Top with water. Add some date sugar to add sweetness to your blend.

ADD YOUR COMMENT: _____

_____

_____

THE W@W FACTOR: *Parsnip* is a root vegetable closely related to carrot and parsley. Its long, tuberous root has cream-colored skin and flesh. The *parsnip* is native to Eurasia, used mainly as sweetener before the arrival in Europe of cane sugar. It is usually cooked but it can also be eaten raw.

Parsnips are rich in potassium, magnesium, phosphorus, manganese and iron. It also contains many vitamins, mainly vitamin C, and fiber together with some protein and folate.

The benefits includes: reduce cholesterol and lower blood pressure which makes it a great allied to the heart; regulates bowel movement and reduce the chances of indigestion, constipation and any other related digestive problems; enhance vision; strengthens bones; reduce diabetes; prevent cancer; boost brain health; improve the immune system and help with weight loss.

The anti-inflammatory properties of Parsnips also help treat many respiratory problems such as asthma. The vitamin C in this vegetable also helps in fighting the respiratory infections and provides relief to people suffering from sinusitis, asthma, bronchitis and other respiratory illnesses.

Stillness in motion   Yes / No

#lunch

lettuce	3 large leaves
banana	1
figs	2
dragon fruit	½
carrot	2 large
celery	2 stalks

HOW TO: juice the carrot and the celery. Wash, chop and add all the other ingredients in the blender

TIPS: if you don't have a juicer, chop one celery and one carrot and add it to the blender (it depend of the speed of your blender, you may need to slightly boil the carrots before to use them). Top with water.

ADD YOUR COMMENT: _____

_____

_____

The Big Bang *Yes / No*

#lunch

apple	2
purple grapes	8
blueberries	2 handful
blue spirulina	1 full tsp
banana	1
purple cabbage	½ cup
blackberries	2 handful
figs	3

HOW TO: juice the apples only. Wash properly all of the ingredients and add it to the blender

TIPS: if you don't have a juicer, simply swap the apples with ½ cup of water and add 1 tsp of date sugar to make it sweet.

ADD YOUR COMMENT: _____

_____

_____

The beginning   Yes / No
                    #lunch

1 small clove of garlic	
beetroot	1
kale	1 handful
pear	1
apple	1
ginger	15 ml
avocado	½

HOW TO: juice the beetroot and the apple. Blend all the ingredients together

TIPS: if the flavour of the garlic is to strong for you, put only half of it in your mix

ADD YOUR COMMENT: _____
_____
_____

One smoothie a day:
As Simple As Two

In this chapter you will find 20 very simple recipes that require only 2 ingredients. Recipes to look at when you fancy a quick, healthy snack or wishing to enjoy simpler tastes. Easy to shop! Easy to make! Easy to drink!

N. 311
Apple and banana
HOW TO: juice 2 apples and blend it with 1 and a ½ banana

N.312
Kiwi and mango
HOW TO: juice 3 kiwis and blended with 1 mango

N.313
Strawberry and carrot
HOW TO: juice 2 large carrots and blended with 6 strawberries

N.314
Cantaloupe melon and papaya
HOW TO: Juice as many pieces of melon as needed to refill 1 cup (~ 1 large slice) and blend it with 1 papaya

N.315
Spinach and pineapple
HOW TO: juice as much pieces of pineapple as needed to refill 1 cup (~ ⅓ of the whole) and blend it with 2 generous handful of spinach

N.316

Beetroot and pear

HOW TO: juice 2 beetroot ad blend it with 2 pears

N.317

Apple and carrot

HOW TO: juice 3 large carrots and blend it with 1 chopped apple

N.318

Dragon fruit and Carrot

HOW TO: Juice 3 large carrots and blend it with one small dragon fruit

N.319

kale and apple

HOW TO: juice 2 apples and blend it with 2 handful of kale

N.320

Strawberry and watermelon

HOW TO: juice the watermelon (¾ cup) and blend it with the strawberries (~7). Or blend both ingredients with a tiny bit of plain water.

N.321

grapefruit and raspberry

HOW TO: juice 1 large grapefruit and blend it with 2 handful of raspberries

N.322

Avocado and apple

HOW TO: juice 2 apples and blend it with 1 avocado

N.323

Carrot and pear

HOW TO: juice as many carrots as needed to fill up your smoothie cup of ¾ . Pour the carrot juice and 1 and ½ large pear in the blender and press START

N.324

Kiwi and pineapple

HOW TO: up to you! You can either juice the 2 ingredients or chop it and place it in the blender with some water. 2 kiwis for ⅓ of pineapple

N.325

Orange and passion fruit

HOW TO: juice 2 and ½ oranges. Scoop the content of one passion fruit out and place it in the blender. Add the juice and blend.

N.326

Lavender tea and blueberries

HOW TO: prepare the tea in advance and let it cool down (add ice cubes if needed). Blend it with a lot but seriously a lot of blueberries. Be generous! a minimum of 2 handful of blueberries required.

N.327

Plums and kiwis

HOW TO: chop 3 kiwis and 2 plums and place it in the blender. Press START. If you rather, you can also juice the kiwis first and then mix it with the plums.

N.328

Blue spirulina and dragon fruit

HOW TO: mix one full teaspoon of spirulina with ¾ cup of water and blend it with your fruit.

N.329

Figs and Mango

HOW TO: Juice 2 mangoes and blend it with 3 figs

N.330

Beetroot and apple

HOW TO: juice two apples and blend it with two beetroot. Or if you prefer, you can juice only all the ingredients and have a refreshing middle day snack.

SMOOTH ME UP... <u>FOR 1 WEEK</u>

Nowadays, there is a great focus on a juice/smoothie diet. Many books have been published about, few documentaries have been filmed, internet is packed with recipes of juices and smoothies ideas to fill your day.

But what are the pros and cons of this type of diet? First of all, let me say that when I use the word 'diet' I do not refer to a meal plan to help you lose weight but rather to a life choice of a overall healthy body/mind system.

Let's start with the CONS. Either if you decide to go for a one day cleanse, three days, one week or a month, the beginning is hard as hell. Of course it depend of body constitution but for the majority of the people the first three days are going to be a real struggle. You will be literally obsessed about food, seeing food everywhere, smelling food, dreaming about food, craving for the most unexpected kind of food ever. You may experience headache, lack of sleep, lack of focus, mood swings, anger, frustration, isolation from the peer group and so on.

This is why I would normally advice to start with a one day detox, maybe to be repeated on a monthly base. Eventually you would then move to a three day detox, to be carry out every three months.

I personally like to do a 7 day detox twice a year, usually after a holiday break when my energy level is high and my mind is still relax and calm. If you do the cleanse during a very busy working period you may have difficulties to get to the end of your journey and experience a deeper lack of energy that may affect the quality of your work. But once again we are all different from one another. Therefore, grab pen and papers, jot down your shopping list and get ready to give it a try and experience the big amount of PROS that comes with it:

- increased focus and concentration
- overall sense of peace
- increase sense of smell and taste
- weight loss
- feeling re-energised
- crave for plant based food instead of junk food
- toxin eliminated for the body
- a clean and irradiate skin
- general feeling of contentment and self appreciation

As you will soon notice, my recipes are quite reach and include a 5 meals plan and this is because my aim is not to bring you to starvation or make you lose 7 kilo in 7 days, this is not the purpose of this book. My goal is to help you discover a better self, a happy and full of energy person that hides behind the stress of the daily life.

In the end of the section I will also illustrate few yoga poses that may help you to keep you dedication intact and your motivation strong and to tone your body whilst detox.

Enjoy!

Antonietta Russo

MONDAY (the excitement begins)

Drink a **hot tea** as you wake up!!!
Suggestion: start your week with a cleansing **fennel tea**

BREAKFAST

N.331   ***THE SWEET START***

Soy yoghurt	half cup
Chia seeds	1 tsp
Oats	1 tbsp
Cocoa	1 tsp
Banana	1 and a half
Oat Milk	half cup
Blueberry	two handfuls

HOW TO: All you need is a blender. Place the banana, blueberries, oats, cocoa, chia seeds, yoghurt and milk inside the blender and press START.
TIPS: add a couple of ice cubes for extra freshness

SNACK

| N.332 | Celery | 3 sticks |
| | Apple | 1 whole |

HOW TO: All you need is a juicer. Place two celery stick, the apple and the remaining celery stick in the juicer and drink up!

TIPS: don't have a juicer? Simple! Place the celery stick in the blender with some still water and a teaspoon of maple syrup or other sweetener you may like to add instead of the apple.

LUNCH

N.333	*THE EASY BEGIN*
Carrot	3 whole
Avocado	1 whole
Spinach	1 handful
Apple	1 whole
Mint	~5 leaves

HOW TO: place the carrots and the apple in the juicer. Place the avocado, mint and spinach in the blender and add the juice of the carrots and apple. Press START

TIPS: which juicer do you have? Be careful! You may need to chop the fruit and vegetables in tiny pieces before to juice.

SNACK

| N.334 | Carrot | 3 whole |
| | Strawberry | ~5 |

HOW TO: place the carrot in the juicer and add the juice to the blender together with the strawberries.

TIPS: would you like to make it even healthier? Why don't you add a half teaspoon of wheatgrass powder to it.

DINNER

N.335	**THE IRON FIST**
Watermelon	1 slice
Cherries	one handful
Mint	~5 leaves
Turmeric	1 tsp
Spinach	one handful

HOW TO: juice the watermelon. Place all the ingredient to the blender and add the watermelon juice before to press START.

TIPS: make sure the cherries are seedless before to place them in the blender

Drink a **hot tea** before to go to sleep!!!

Suggestion: why don't try a **camomile tea** for a better night sleep

TUESDAY (I feel the struggle)

Drink a **hot tea** as you wake up!!!
Suggestion: go for a **green tea** to irradiate your skin

BREAKFAST

N.336   **I am vanilla!**

Cinnamon	1 tsp
Vanilla soy milk	1 cup
Vanilla soy yoghurt	half a cup
Banana	1 whole
Cherry	1 handful
Maple	1 tsp

HOW TO: place all the ingredient in the blender and press START
TIPS: place the cinnamon and the maple halfway through in the blender to avoid that the powder will stick to the blander

SNACK

N.337	Apple	2 whole
	Ice cubes	2

HOW TO: place the apples in the juicer and then move it to the blender adding a couple of ice cubes for freshness
TIPS: avoid to drink apple juice bought from a store because it always contains additive and preservative that your body doesn't need and it only contribute to unhealthy habits.

LUNCH

N.338   **THE MIX THAT WORKS!**

Broccoli   half cup
Cashew nuts soaked   half cup
Almond Milk   1 cup
Basil   ~3 leaves
Peanut Butter   1 tbsp

HOW TO: place all the ingredient in a blender and press START
TIPS: place the peanut butter half way into the blender to avoid to stick to the bottom.

SNACK

N.339   Spinach   1 handful
               Carrot   2 whole
               Apple   1 whole

HOW TO: place the carrot and apple in the juicer and then bland together with the spinach
TIPS: add some spirulina powder for a boost of energy

DINNER

N.340   **The Citrus**
Lime   half
Lemon   half
Carrot   3 whole
Spinach   one handful
Kale   one handful
Pear   1 whole
Grapefruit   1 whole

HOW TO: juice the carrots, grapefruit, lemon and lime before to add its juice to the blender together with the rest of the ingredient
TIPS: make sure the pear is chopped and all the seeds are removed before to place it in the blender

Drink a **hot tea** before to go to sleep!!!
Suggestion: why don't try a **red berry tea** to awaken your sense of smell

WEDNESDAY (Help!!!I want to eat...but I won't!)

Drink a **hot tea** as you wake up!!!
Suggestion: go for a **lemon tea** to purify your intestine

BREAKFAST:
N.341   **THE LONG DAY SOLUTION**

Coffee powder	1 tsp
Cacao powder	1 tsp
Banana	1 and a half
Soy Milk	1 and a half cup
Crumbled biscuits	half cup

HOW TO: place the banana first in the blender, add the crumbled biscuits, the coffee and cacao powders and the milk before to press START.
TIPS: do you know that you can also eat a smoothie? Why don't you place your mix in a bowl and add some dark chocolate shaving as topping

SNACK
N.342

Apple	2 whole
Banana	1 whole

HOW TO: juice the apple first and then bland together with the banana
TIPS: why don't spice it up a little with few drops of freshly squeezed ginger added to the mix

LUNCH
N.343   **THE HALF WAY THROUGH**

Orange	2 whole
Avocado	1 whole
Mint	~5 leaves
Carrot	2 whole
Ice	3 ice cubes

HOW TO: juice the carrot and the orange. Place in the blender the ice with the avocado and mint and add the juice before to press START.

TIPS: make sure the orange is peeled before to juice it

SNACK

N.344	Carrot	2 whole
	Beetroot	1 whole

HOW TO: place in the juicer 1 carrot, 1 beetroot and the second carrot to mix the flavour.

TIPS: wash and peel the beetroot properly before to juice

DINNER

N.345	**THE MORE THE BETTER**
Tomato	1 whole
Fennel	half
Yellow bell pepper	half
Beetroot	1 whole
Apple	2 whole

HOW TO: juice the beetroot and the apples before to add them to the blender with the rest of the mix.

TIPS: you can actually juice all of the ingredients. It's up to you opt for a smooth dinner or a light juice. The third day is usually the hardest one so go easy on yourself and blend it all up. Feeling famishing? Add a banana or half of an avocado to the mix for a more fulfilling taste

Drink a **hot tea** before to go to sleep!!!

Suggestion: why don't try a **white tea** to warm your body up before to slide under the duvet.

THURSDAY (I am the queen/king of the day)

Drink a **hot tea** as you wake up!!!
Suggestion: go for a **mint tea** to embrace that feeling of being unstoppable that usually arise on the 4th day

BREAKFAST

N.346	**I'm going NUTS**
Walnuts	3 whole or one full tbsp of crushed walnut
Peanut Butter	1 tbsp
Almond Milk	1 cup
Cashew nuts	1 tbsp
Almond Yoghurt	1/2 cup
Banana	1 whole

HOW TO: is better if you soaked the cashew nuts overnight for a creamier taste. Place the banana first and then all the other ingredient.
TIPS: if you don't have the time to soak the cashew you can bring them to boil for a 15 minutes time.

SNACK

N.347	Coconut Water	1 cup
	Banana	½

HOW TO: only use the blender. Place the banana and the coconut water together and press START.
TIPS: feeling really hungry? Add an extra banana to the blend.

LUNCH

N.348	**The all green**
Spinach	1 handful
Kale	1 handful
Cucumber	1 whole
Celery	3 sticks
Kiwi	1 whole
Parsley	~6 leaves

HOW TO: juice the medium sized cucumber and the celery sticks. Add all the other ingredient to the blender with the juice and press START.

TIPS: if you like it sweeter add an extra kiwi to the mix.

SNACK

N.349	Carrot	4 large
	Blueberry	1 handful

HOW TO: juice the carrots and blend them with the blueberry

TIPS: to bitter? Add half apple to sweet it up

DINNER

N.350	**Sunglasses Needs**
Passion fruit	1
Papaya	1
Honey dew melon	2 slices
Pineapple	½
Banana	1

HOW TO: juice the pineapple and the melon and add the other ingredient to blend

TIPS: cut out the central part of the pineapple: is bitter and not really good to juice!

Drink a **hot tea** before to go to sleep!!!

Suggestion: why don't try a **vanilla tea** to share the bedtime with.

FRIDAY (It's getting easier!)

Drink a **hot tea** as you wake up!!!
Suggestion: go for a **black tea** of your choice to kick start your day

BREAKFAST
N.351   **Breakfast we go!**

Oats	1 tbsp
Cocoa	1 tbsp
Oats Milk	1-1/2 cup
Banana	1 whole
Mix Berry	1 handful

HOW TO: place the banana and berries first in the blender and then add all the other ingredient
TIPS: you can either use fresh berry or frozen berries

SNACK
N.352

Carrot	2 whole
Apple	1 whole
Orange	1 whole

HOW TO: juice all the ingredients
TIPS: add ice for freshness

LUNCH
N.353   **The reach beet!**

Beetroot	2 whole
Celery	1 stick
Mint	~5 leaves
Carrot	2 whole
Avocado	½
Banana	1/2

HOW TO: juice the beetroot, carrot and celery. Add all the other ingredient to the blender and press START.

TIPS: add a wheatgrass powder to feel more energized

SNACK

N.354	Beetroot	2
	Apple	1

HOW TO: you only need the juicer!

TIPS: remember to wash your juicer straight after the use for a easy cleaning solution

DINNER

N.355	**The big cleanse**	
Watermelon	1 slice	
Honey dew melon	1 slice	
Cantaloupe melon	1 slice	

HOW TO: you only need the juicer!

TIPS: don't have a juicer? Chop the fruits and blended with a little bit of water.

Drink a **hot tea** before to go to sleep!!!

Suggestion: why don't try a relaxing **passion flower leaf tea** to induce really sweet dreams!

SATURDAY (who is the champion?)

Drink a **hot tea** as you wake up!!!
Suggestion: go for a **liquorice tea** to flavour your way through the day

BREAKFAST
N.356   **The morning bomb**

Peanut butter	1 tbsp
Oats	1 tbsp
Almond yoghurt	2 tbsp
Chia seeds	1 tsp
Almond Milk	½ cup
Banana	2

HOW TO: place the milk, yoghurt and banana as based for the blender and add on top the leftover ingredient.
TIPS: try to let the chia seed soak with the yoghurt or milk for ~30 minutes before to blend for an improved taste

SNACK
N.357

Fennel	1 small
Celery	3 sticks

HOW TO: juice both ingredient or chop it and bland with little water
TIPS: too spicy? Add half of an apple to sweet it all up.

LUNCH
N.358   **The hunger solution**

Beetroot	1
Kiwi	1
Carrots	5
Avocado	1
Mint	~5 leaves

Spinach   1 handful

HOW TO: juice the carrots and beetroot and then blend it with the rest of the ingredient
TIPS: add a mixed protein powder to have that extra boost of energy

SNACK:
N.359

          Cucumber   1
          Mint   ~5 leaves

HOW TO: place the cucumber in the juicer and then blend it together with the mint
TIPS: option to cut the cucumber in small parts and blended with the mint and a little bit of water

DINNER
N.360   <u>**The purifying sip**</u>
Green tea   1 and a half cup
Lemon zest   of half of a lemon
Avocado   ½
Blueberry   1/2 cup

HOW TO: soak a green tea bag in a 1/2 cup of hot water, remove the tea bag and add one more cup of cold water. Place it in the blender together with the rest of the ingredients and
TIPS: opt for a little lemon juice if you like

Drink a **hot tea** before to go to sleep!!!
Suggestion: time for a **hot water with fresh ginger**. Add a drop of maple syrup if you like.

SUNDAY(I am the best I ever been!)

Drink a **hot tea** as you wake up!!!
Suggestion: choose your favourite tea to enjoy every moment of this last fantastic day.

BREAKFAST

N.361	The coolest morning
Raspberry	1/2 cup
Yoghurt	1/2 cup
Ice	3 cubes
Celery	4 sticks
Water	1/2 cup

HOW TO: juice the celeries and then place all the ingredient in the blender and press START
TIPS: add less water or not water for a thicker smoothie option

SNACK

N.362

Kiwi	4 whole

HOW TO: peel the fruit and place it in the juicer.
TIPS: don't have a juicer? Chop the fruit and place it in the blender with little water

LUNCH

N.363	The one and for all
Broccoli	1 handful
Spinach	1 handful
Beetroot	4
Parsley	~5 leaves
Avocado	1

HOW TO: juice the beetroot and add all the ingredient to the blender

TIPS: scare it will taste to bitter? Reduce the amount of beetroot and add some plain water instead. Option to also add a drop of maple syrup.

SNACK
N.364

Apple	2
Mango	1

HOW TO: juice it all up!
TIPS: feeling hungry? Add a banana to the blend

DINNER
N.365   **The tropical**

Coconut water	1 cup
Pineapple	½
Mango	1

HOW TO: chop the fruit and mix it all in the blender
TIPS: remove the central part of the pineapple to avoid excess of bitterness

Drink a **hot tea** before to go to sleep!!!
Suggestion: opt for a chamomile tea for a deep and dreamless well deserved dream

WELL DONE!!!!
How do you feel? How many great ideas your mind free of toxin has developed? How is your skin looking? How does your mood going?
Write down the ups and down of the week and underlying your greatest achievements.

Keep adding a juice to your meal time to time to don't lose this great conquer!

YOGA FOR HEALTH

As a certified yoga teacher I felt, in writing this book, to be a necessity to add this short session. Often people struggle in life, struggle to maintain a healthy eating habit, struggle to face the smallest challenges at work and in the personal relationships because most basically we don't breath in the right way. Oh yeah my lovely readers, is simple as breath in and out, inhale and exhale. In this sense, yoga is for everybody, this session of the book is for everybody. It is a session that deserve to be read **if you believe to be worthy of happiness in your life**. If you most simply need help to get through your weekly smoothie challenge or most intensively you feel the need of a guide for your daily struggle, whatever they are: depression, anxiety, social awkwardness, anger, shyness, panic attack or on a more physically point of view if you lack core strength, if you lack of focus and peace in your mind... this short little session is here for you.

We will explore together how to breath properly (you may be doing it right already, therefore carry on or you may need to follow my suggestions) and we will explore few yoga asanas (poses) to strengthen the core and increase the stillness of the mind in order to gain contentment of our present and strength to face our future. Are very simple, sometimes, incredibly obvious asanas....therefore, no excuses!

Steady, ready, go!

Asana 1: **crossed leg pose**

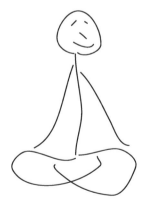

<u>First of all, we breathe!</u>

Choose a comfortable sitting pose. It can be on the floor, crossed legs, or on a block, or even on a chair. If you prefer, you may also stand if for any health related reason your body doesn't allow you to sit comfortably.

My personal choice is to sit on the floor, placing a short block under my sit bones in order to reduce the pressure in the knee joints as I cross my legs and remove curves in the spine.

If you like to sit on a block, like me, but the crossed legs add to much tension to your knee area you have many options...create a butterfly shape with your legs by join the soles of the feet together and dropping the knee out to the side...make sure there is quite a lot of space between the feet and the centre of your body (we do not want to add unnecessary tension).

Option 2: bend the knees, knees pointing towards the ceiling, soles of the feet on the floor, halfway close to your buttocks.

Option 3: leave the legs straight on the floor

Remove the flashy part of your buttocks out of the way and make sure you are sitting with a nice, long and straight spine.

Roll the shoulders up, back and down a couple of times and then push them down and back, leaving your chest open and the heart shining.

Chin slightly tuck towards the chest, neck long, growing through the crown of your head.

1} Place one hand under the belly button, one hand above the belly button.

Take a deep breath in and as you inhale push the belly out. Allow the belly to be fill with air and press the hands away. As your inhale becomes deeper and longer you should notice the thumb of one hand and the index of the other hand moving away from each other.

Begin to count your inhale: 1-2-3-4. You may notice that in the beginning you can only breathe in for one count and this is fine...try to add an extra count if you can!

Maybe your breath is 6 or 7 counts, or more...knowing how you breathing is so so so important.

Now do the same thing with the exhale. As you exhale, push the belly in, allow the fingers to touch each other and your mind to count the length of the breathe.

Here we go: **10 deep breath in, push the belly out, and 10 slow breath out, squeeze the belly in**.

2} Slide the hands on each side of the rib cage and bring your focus to the middle part of your torso. Inhale and push the ribs out to the side, allowing your hands to expand side to side. Exhale and drop the ribs in, allowing your hands to squeeze.

Count the length of your breath and proceed for 10 times

3} Slide the hands on top of your chest: one hand on top of the other and bring your focus to this area.

As you inhale lift the chest and push the chest into your hands. As you exhale, drop the chest.

Count the length of each inhale and exhale and repeat for 10 times.

If you are in a crossed legs position, swap the cross of the legs and release the arms and hands down. Place the top of the hands over the knees with the palms face up. Take a long inhale and push the belly out, keep breathing in and expand the rib cages, keep breathing in and lift the chest.

Exhale and drop the chest first, keep exhaling and squeeze the rib cage, keep exhaling and bring the tummy in.

Repeat for 5 times...if you can get to 10! No need to count at this point.

How can this help you?

In order to be able to perform this simple but intense practice you need to maintain your focus at all times, otherwise you will go back immediately to your shallow breath. Increases your focus, increases your will power and enhances your mood. And, on top of it, we are warming up and strengthening our abdominal muscles, getting ready for the rest of the practice.

If you don't have much time in the morning do only this exercise. It will take only 3 minutes of your time!

Asana 2: **seated side bend**

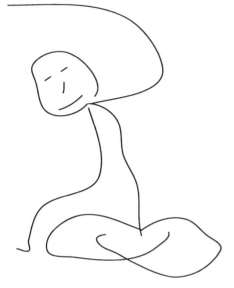

Stay in your crossed leg or sitting pose of your choice. Place the right hand down, close to your right hip. Bend slightly the right elbow. Stretch the left arm over the head and slowly move the left hand toward the right side. It's a side bend which help to stretch the lateral of the abdominal wall, making your core strong but released from any tension. Keep your gaze on the floor in front of your or if it's ok with your neck come to look toward your left fingertips.

Take 5 deep breath!

Option to move straight to the other side, option to do circles with your arm. Begin with a couple of small circles and get to very big circle where also your torso is moving...but not your sit bones (your lower body is as steady as it can be). Circle for 10: exhale when you circle the arm down, inhale when you circle the arm up.

As you end your last circle, drop the left hand next to the left hip, bend slightly the left elbow. Rise the right arm over the head and slightly to the left. Fix your gaze and breath for 5. Add the circle if you like an extra opening of the side of the abdominal wall. Remember not to move the lower body but if the sitting position start to become uncomfortable give a little shake to your leg and then come back.

Asana 3: **seated twist**

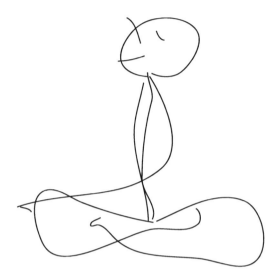

With the lower body still in the same position, place now the right hand on the outside of the left knee and the left hand behind your body (ideally behind the sacrum) have a soft bend in the left elbow. Take a deep breath in and straighten the spine, exhale and begin to look back. Try to push the left shoulder as back as you can. Have the chin slightly tuck toward the left shoulder. Fix the gaze. Take 3 deep breath in here. At the third exhale release and go for the other side. With this asana, we improve the focus and willpower while stretching the abdominal wall from side to side.

Asana 4: **cat and cow**

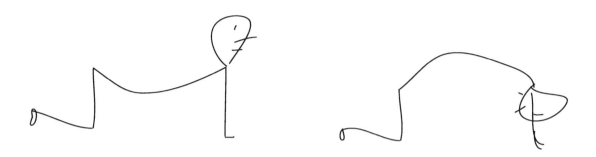

Organize your body on a kneeling position. Hands and knees on the floor/yoga mat. Place the hands right under the shoulders and the knees right under the hips. Check that the hands are shoulders distance apart and that the knees and feet are hip width apart. Have your spine completely straight as you contract the abdominal muscles and push the chest slightly in, in order to open the space between the shoulder blades.

Once settle, take a deep breath in, while dropping the belly down, arching the spine and lifting the gaze toward the ceiling (check with your neck how far back is happy to go).

Exhale and curve the spine while the eyes come and look down between the legs.

Repeat for 10

With this asanas you will not only massage the vertebrae (goodbye lower back pain) but you will also constantly contracting and expanding the abs making your abdominal walls strong and flexible.

Asana 5: **low launch with twist**

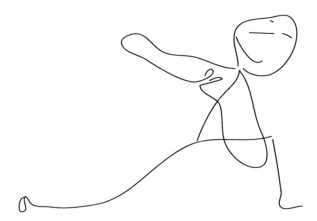

Step the right foot in between your hands, push the hips forward and allow them to sink as far down into the ground as they feel to go. Keep the back foot stable. Lift the torso and then place the left elbow on the outside of the right knee, join the arms together in a prayer position and let the right elbows pointing up towards the ceiling. Remember to keep the shoulder relax and far away from the ears. Look towards your top elbows if its ok for your balance and your neck, otherwise keep your eyes fix on the floor. A quick look to your knee to ensure that is right above the ankle and not pushed forward.
Take 5 deep breath.
This asana helps massage the internal organs, releasing from lower back tension and stretch the abdominal wall from side to side

After your 5th breath come back to centre with your torso and then release the hands flat on the floor, one on each side of the front foot. Lift the back knee and swing with the entire body back and forth, pushing the shoulders and the heel front and back in order to stretch the lower body before to move to the next asana.

Asana 6: **cactus arms in high launch**

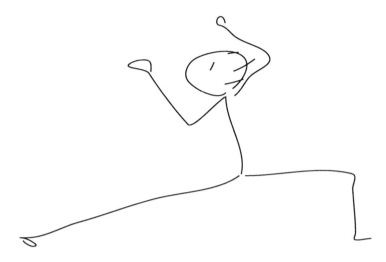

Keep the back knee still lifted, find stability and lift the torso up (option to drop the back knee down if your balance is out of order for the day!). The front knee is still bend and stuck above the ankle. The back heel is lifted while the toes are pushing down into the ground.

Push the abdomen as back as you can while straighten the arms up with an inhale, look up and exhale bending the elbows in a cactus shape. Check that the elbows are shoulders height and that the elbows are push as back as possible. You should feel the shoulder blades squeezing on the back of your body. Also try to have the hands stuck right over the elbow at all times. In this way we are stretching and expanding the entire abdomen.

Hold it for 5 breath.

Be mindful not to tense the shoulders and neck but to leave lot of space between the shoulders and the ears.

Asana 7: **warrior 2**

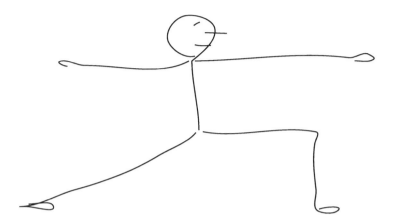

And we couldn't leave a warrior pose out of the picture, am I right? Let's explore warrior 2!
It is time for the back heel to reach for the floor, having the toes pointing a 45 degrees angle. Let the hips be open and looking toward the left side of the room. Arms are in a T-shape, shoulder pressing down while arms and finger are very active and engaged. Fix your gaze toward the front finger tips. Front knee is still bend and still stuck over the ankle.
Tilt the pelvic floor under while squeezing the belly in.
Take 5 deep breath in.

Well done!

Asana 8: **triangle pose**

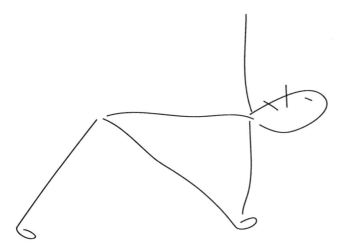

We finally straighten that front leg, maintaining a soft bend in the knee in order not to lock your leg. Back leg and hips are still in the same position. Upper body still the same.

Push the right arm as forward as you can, before to lower the fingertips toward the right ankle. Maintain the arms still in a T-shape and only if it's ok for your neck and balance come to look towards your top fingertips. Keep pushing the belly in while taking 5 deep breath.

Asana 9: **Downward Facing Dog**

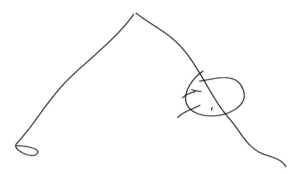

Time for our first Downward Facing Dog. Place the left palm flat on the floor, right palm too!
Step the right foot back to join the left and let them be hip distance apart. Hands are shoulders distance apart. Hips as high as possible. Try to create a revolved V-shape. Try to push the heels as close to the floor as possible: they don't have to touch the floor but in this way you will allow the back of the body to extend. Contract the abdominal muscle at all times.
Hold for 5 breath
Option 1 bend the knees one at the time while up in your down dog...it makes it easier to hold
Option 2 drop your knees down and find a child pose: knees together with the hands pointing back along your body or knees wide apart with only the toes touching and the arms stretching forward.

P.s. the best way to understand if in Down Dog your hands and feet are at the right distance is to move forward in high plank, check that the wrists are right under the shoulders and then push the hips back up.

Asana 10: **halfway lift**

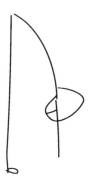 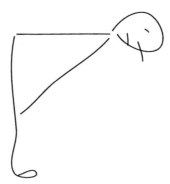

Step or walk the feet towards your hands. Feet hip distance apart to begin with. Swing the arms from side to side, simply to realize any tension you may have in you upper body. Come back to center with your arms. Allow the big toes to touch, heels slightly apart. Inhale, bring the palms to rest on the thigh while the spine is halfway lift, straight with the crown of the head reaching toward the front of the room.

Move in this motion for 10 breaths: exhale, drop the arms down, head down and spine curved; inhale, rise the palms on top of the thigh, just above the knees, flatten the spine.

End with the exhale in which your arms are dropping down.

Asana 11: **standing side bend**

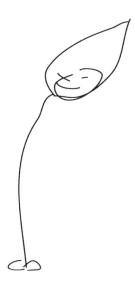

Keep your spine curve and abdomen contract and begin to unroll one vertebrae at the time while lifting the torso up to stand. Keep lifting the arms over the head. Allow your fingers to be engages while reaching for the ceiling. Stretch your abdomen from bottom to top.

Use the right hand to grasp the left wrist and bend to the right side as you exhale. Inhale back to center, change the grasp of your hands, exhale inge toward the left.

Repeat for 5.

Asana 12: **Tree pose**

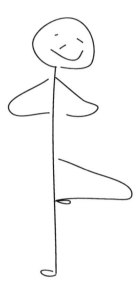

Tree pose. Release the hands on top of the hips. Shift the weight over to the left leg. Inhale and begin to lift the right foot to touch the left ankle. Maybe it may go all the way up on the inside of the left thigh. If it's okay for your balance, hands can join in a prayer pose. Contract the abdomen at all times and hold for 5 breath. Have a sense of uplift accompany you during this journey.

Go for the other side

Release legs and arms, drop the chin close to the chest and begin to curve your spine, making your way down. Bend the knees if you need too in order to flatten your palms on the floor. Step the right foot back, right knees drops.
Repeat Asanas 5-6-7-8-9 on the other side

Asana 13: **Camel pose**

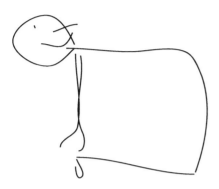

From your Downward Dog, drop the knees down to the floor/yoga mat.

Tuck the toes under, lift the torso and place your hand on the lower back finger pointing up (if this option is available for you today). Chin tuck. Take a deep breath in, exhale begin to move the shoulder back, arching the spine. Hold for one breath and then come back up and we do this 2 more times. If you like, and your vertebrae are happy with it, while arching back realise the fingers to reach for the heels while pushing the hips forward. Hold your last one for a top of 5 breaths.

Move into child pose for a little rest

Asana 14: **Boat pose**

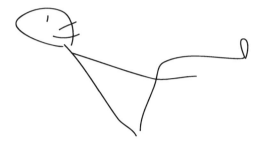

Come to sit and find your boat by balancing on the seat bones. Place your hands on the back of the thighs and begin to lift one foot at the time. Create a 90 degrees angle with your knees and straighten the arms along the legs, parallel to the floor. Option to keep the hands behind the thighs and only lifting one foot at the time off the floor. The more you hold the pose the more you will feel your abs shaking

Asana 15: **Revolved table top**

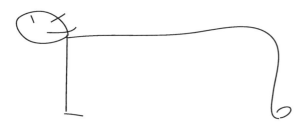

Place your feet down, still halfway close to your buttock. Palm down and back with the fingertips pointing toward your body. Inhale and lift the hips. Hold for 5 deep, steady breathes.

Asana 16: **Head to Knees**

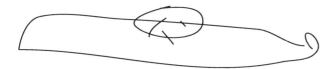

Slowly release the hips down and straighten the legs. Take a deep inhale while lifting the arms over the head with a long vertebral column. Exhale and fold the torso towards your legs while reaching the fingers towards the outer edge of the feet.
In this pose be mindful not to lock the knees but always maintaining a soft bend. Also, you don't have to touch the feet, more easily just hold onto the ankles or calves.
Listen to your body!

RELEASE your body from the previous asana.

Cross your legs and place again a block under your buttock. Repeat asana 3 (side to side twist), and asana 2 (side bend).

Exchange cross of the legs. *Place the palms of your hands on top of the knees, locking the positive energy within your body.* Close your eyes for just a moment and bring your focus on the centre of your body, your abdominal wall. Picture a ball of fire, a red little ball becoming bigger and bigger as you inhale and exhale. It become so big that at a certain point your body cannot longer contain it. Picture this ball shooting out your abdomen, reaching the middle of the room and exploding in billions of spectacular fireworks.

It's amazing

All the tension as just left your body and you are light and carefree and ready to face a new wonderful day

with love and light

Namaste'

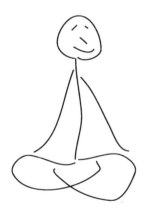

I hope you guys have enjoyed reading this book as much as I did writing it.
Don't put it in on the shelf but keep it always with you, available. You never know when the need of getting a
blended meal is going to struck you. And when that moment comes, I will be here gifting you with tasty ideas
for every palate.

I wish you all a magical, healthy life

Antonietta Russo

It's on you!

Enough of following other people recipes, it's time for you to create your own mix. Be the artist! Be the creator! Be the giver of life! This space is for you: have fun by mixing and matching the ingredients on your cupboard and when you'll find something that works well don't just forget about it but write it down in this special recipes section.

1.   NAME of the SMOOTHIE_____

ingredients list   _____

                     _____

                     _____

                     _____

                     _____

                     _____

                     _____

                     _____

                     _____

how to proceed: _____

_____

_____

_____

_____

2.   NAME of the SMOOTHIE_____

ingredients list   _____

                     _____

                     _____

                     _____

                     _____

                     _____

_____
_____

how to proceed: _____
_____
_____
_____
_____

3.   NAME of the SMOOTHIE_____

ingredients list   _____
                    _____
                    _____
                    _____
                    _____
                    _____
                    _____
                    _____
                    _____

how to proceed: _____
_____
_____
_____
_____

4.   NAME of the SMOOTHIE_____

ingredients list   _____

                      _____

                      _____

                      _____

                      _____

                      _____

                      _____

                      _____

                      _____

how to proceed: _____

_____

_____

_____

_____

5.   NAME of the SMOOTHIE_____

ingredients list   _____

                      _____

                      _____

                      _____

                      _____

                      _____

                      _____

                      _____

                      _____

how to proceed: _____

_____

_____

_____

_____

6.   NAME of the SMOOTHIE_____

ingredients list   _____

                    _____

                    _____

                    _____

                    _____

                    _____

                    _____

                    _____

                    _____

how to proceed: _____
_____
_____
_____
_____

7.   NAME of the SMOOTHIE_____

ingredients list   _____

                    _____

                    _____

                    _____

                    _____

                    _____

                    _____

                    _____

how to proceed: _____
_____
_____
_____
_____

8.   NAME of the SMOOTHIE_____

ingredients list   _____

                    _____

                    _____

                    _____

                    _____

                    _____

                    _____

                    _____

                    _____

how to proceed: _____

_____

_____

_____

_____

9.   NAME of the SMOOTHIE_____

ingredients list   _____

                    _____

                    _____

                    _____

                    _____

                    _____

                    _____

                    _____

                    _____

how to proceed: _____

_____

_____

_____

_____

10.   NAME of the SMOOTHIE_____

ingredients list   _____

                     _____

                     _____

                     _____

                     _____

                     _____

                     _____

                     _____

                     _____

how to proceed: _____

_____

_____

_____

_____

the W@W Factor list:

1.	acai	smoothie n. 157
2.	agave syrup	smoothie n. 161
3.	almond	smoothie n. 181
4.	apple	smoothie n. 174
5.	aubergine	smoothie n. 271
6.	avocado	smoothie n. 2
7.	banana	smoothie n. 206
8.	basil	smoothie n. 164
9.	beetroot	smoothie n. 173
10.	bell pepper	smoothie n. 180
11.	black pepper	smoothie n. 54
12.	blueberry	smoothie n. 197
13.	broccoli	smoothie n. 194
14.	cabbage	smoothie n. 150
15.	cantaloupe melon	smoothie n. 166
16.	carrot	smoothie n. 63
17.	cashew nut	smoothie n. 202
18.	celery	smoothie n. 12
19.	cherry	smoothie n. 205
20.	chestnut	smoothie n. 162
21.	chia seed	smoothie n. 154
22.	chickpea	smoothie n. 196
23.	cinnamon	smoothie n. 177
24.	cocoa bean	smoothie n. 195
25.	coconut	smoothie n. 115
26.	coffee	smoothie n. 169
27.	coriander	smoothie n. 226
28.	cranberry	smoothie n. 158
29.	cucumber	smoothie n. 172
30.	date	smoothie n. 117
31.	dragon fruit	smoothie n. 296
32.	fennel	smoothie n. 198
33.	fig	smoothie n. 189
34.	flaxseed	smoothie n. 147

35.	garlic	smoothie n. 143
36.	ginger	smoothie n. 144
37.	goji berry	smoothie n. 124
38.	golden syrup	smoothie n. 266
39.	granola	smoothie n. 168
40.	grapefruit	smoothie n. 74
41.	green tea	smoothie n. 170
42.	hemp	smoothie n. 151
43.	kale	smoothie n. 163
44.	kiwifruit	smoothie n. 193
45.	lavender	smoothie n. 149
46.	lemon	smoothie n. 203
47.	lentil	smoothie n. 204
48.	lettuce	smoothie n. 178
49.	lime	smoothie n. 190
50.	liquorice	smoothie n. 254
51.	maca	smoothie n. 146
52.	mandarin	smoothie n. 165
53.	mango	smoothie n. 130
54.	maple syrup	smoothie n. 160
55.	matcha tea	smoothie n. 171
56.	mint	smoothie n. 114
57.	oat	smoothie n. 179
58.	olive	smoothie n. 159
59.	orange	smoothie n. 142
60.	papaya	smoothie n. 182
61.	parsley	smoothie n. 145
62.	parsnip	smoothie n. 307
63.	passion fruit	smoothie n. 136
64.	peach	smoothie n. 153
65.	pear	smoothie n. 45
66.	pineapple	smoothie n. 188
67.	pomegranate	smoothie n. 264
68.	potato	smoothie n. 255
69.	prune	smoothie n. 152
70.	Pumpkin	smoothie n. 133

71.	radish	smoothie n. 251
72.	raspberry	smoothie n. 187
73.	rice	smoothie n. 242
74.	rocket	smoothie n. 167
75.	soya bean	smoothie n. 139
76.	spinach	smoothie n. 116
77.	spirulina	smoothie n. 148
78.	strawberries	smoothie n. 59
79.	tahini sauce	smoothie n. 209
80.	tomato	smoothie n. 127
81.	turmeric	smoothie n. 24
82.	vanilla	smoothie n. 17
83.	wasabi	smoothie n. 223
84.	water	smoothie n. 199
85.	watermelon	smoothie n. 212
86.	zucchini	smoothie n. 237

Acknowledgments

A deep thank you goes to all the people that have been supporting me in this past few months while creating this book. I don't need to mention them because I always try to tell them in my everyday life how special they are for me and how much value they are adding to my existence.

A special acknowledgement goes to you! To you that have just bought my book, our book. Because thanks to you I can continue to follow my passion for writing, my passion for healthy living, my passion for helping others by modifying the little everyday habits.

Thank you for helping me and thank you for allow me to help you.

May the sunlight always shine your way through each and every breath you are gifted with.

Antonietta Russo

Printed in Poland
by Amazon Fulfillment
Poland Sp. z o.o., Wrocław